PSYCHO-ONCOLOGY, HYPNOSIS AND PSYCHOSOMATIC HEALING IN CANCER

Francisco O. Valenzuela Ph.D.

Trafford rev. 03/27/2015

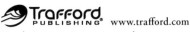 www.trafford.com

North America & international
toll-free: 1 888 232 4444 (USA & Canada)
fax: 812 355 4082

This book is dedicated to Matilde, my wife and mentor, to our parents, to our clients and finally, to Clarita Venegas, my childhood teacher, who told me that the brain, not money, is what sets apart one individual from another.

Contents

PREFACE

This was our first trip to Boston, Massachusetts.

On a damp October day my wife Matilde and I walked the narrow and winding streets, not knowing where the Longwood Medical Centre area was located. Our destination was the Joseph Martin Conference building, adjacent to the Harvard Medical School.

Five months ago, we decided to enrol in a continuing education seminar aptly named "The Revolutionary Practice of Mind-body Medicine," sponsored by the Benson-Henry Institute for Mind-body Medicine at the Harvard Medical School. It was going to be an exciting and exhausting set of ten days of studying in a program directed by Dr. Herbert Benson himself.

To us it was analogous to climbing Mt. Everest.

It was an emotional moment and a long way from my hometown of Traiguen—region of the Araucania, in the southern part of Chile—to Boston, Massachusetts, the place where I was going to find the elusive scientific evidence that, in my opinion, my clinical approach needed.

It was a very personal endeavour, for none of my clients demanded from me an evidence-based dissertation on the Psychobiology of Mind-body Healing to establish a connection between science and my work as a clinical-medical hypnotherapist and psycho-oncologist.

They only wanted a professional to provide them with hope and encouragement, which was what they needed to tackle their sickness.

Our travel agent (who apparently never visited Boston) was of the impression that Harvard Plaza was the place we were supposed to go; therefore she found us a hotel close to the Plaza in Medford, a town within a town in Boston.

Big mistake! The Longwood Medical Centre was about one hour and fifteen minutes from our hotel.

One block from the hotel, we took a bus to Davis Square then a red "T" train to Park Station. We walked up and down through a series of stairs and platforms to finally find the green "D" train to Longwood station. Our logic told us that the Longwood Medical Centre must be in Longwood.

Another big mistake! Longwood Medical Centre was in the vicinity of a different line: the "E" train to Heath. It was already 8:00 AM. We were supposed to be at the Joseph Martin Conference Centre at 8:30 AM.

We did not have a clear idea where we were. We saw a young lady approaching us, and we asked her in our best English about the whereabouts of the conference centre. We produced our map, and she responded in perfect Spanish that we had to cross the tracks over to the other side of the park.

We were about twenty blocks from our destination, and the young lady was from Ecuador. This was our first encounter with a multitude of Spanish-speaking people, for in Boston, Spanish is like a second language.

In this cloudy and humid day we resolved to walk the distance, hoping that the rain would show mercy on these stranded Latino-Canadians. We decided to enjoy the walk.

At 9:00 AM, we arrived at the Conference Centre—the starting place of our foray into the world of Dr. Herbert Benson, a physician already in the history of Medicine.

It was Matilde's brilliant idea to rehearse the trip; for it was Sunday, the day before the initiation of the seminar.

Thank goodness for female intuition and foresight!

We learned that there was another green train going to Longwood Medical Centre, leaving us only three blocks—not twenty—from our objective.

We also discovered the "Charlie Pass," a card that gave us access to all the trains and buses of Boston and those of the surrounding area. It was only $15.00 per person, and it became our ticket to the grand tour of Boston. The "Charlie Pass" became our lucky charm.

Now we were ready for our adventure!

I found my evidence on the first day of classes. Moreover, I found people that were passionate about fully empowering and incorporating their clients into the healing process.

I validated my conviction that trance is the appropriate vehicle to go beyond the Relaxation Response and into the information contained in the unconscious mind and embodied as state-dependent learning and behavior, information which supports the state-bound blueprints for sickness.

I felt that I found the pot of gold at the end of my rainbow.

INTRODUCTION

<u>HEALING IS ABOUT ATTITUDE!</u>

A remarkable experience happened on the evening of March 26, 2013.

Matilde and I attended a calligraphy course offered by Steven Aung MD, PhD, OMD, FAAFP.

Dr. Aung is a pioneer in the integration of western, traditional Chinese, and complementary medicine. He is a gentle, kind, and compassionate physician and artist who integrates many activities into medicine— one of them being calligraphy, which in his opinion is a most spiritual experience.

While delivering his first lesson in an almost packed classroom in the Faculty of Medicine at the University of Alberta in Edmonton, he stated that concentration and connection with our heart is an indispensable condition to do calligraphy. He positioned himself in front of his demonstration table with his legs separated as in a combat position. He grabbed his brush, and with a martial arts scream "Haaa!" Dr. Aung stroked the first line on his rice paper.

After the initial confusion, he explained that calligraphy is about concentration, connection with the self, and attitude. The line has to be firm but gentle, and there is to be determination and a proper body balance; for this is what makes a calligrapher good. He added that to create an integral self, compassion and love has to be added to the work; for love and compassion permeates everything in the universe.

It was, in my opinion, a perfect metaphor to illustrate the difference between a healer and a practitioner.

A practitioner works in an impartial and nonpartisan fashion on the expressions of the sickness—solving, if possible, the symptoms that characterize it and exhibiting no emotion with only science driving his work.

A healer, with his emotions in perfect balance, works with the whole person's fears, emotions, spirituality, and dreams—adding to the equation hope, love, and compassion with all of it shrouded in a fearless attitude of concentration and determination to awaken the warrior hidden inside the client's bodymind, and further adding to this equation his scientific acumen.

It is the "Haaa!" that makes the line defined.

It is amazing what you can learn in a calligraphy class with Dr. Aung!

At times serendipity places me in the right place to find the answers to not-so-clearly-formulated questions while searching for ways to help my wife to deal with her cancer and her vanished well-being, health, and happiness. The place was the American Institute of Hypnotherapy (AIH); and one of the instructors in the roster was Bruce Lipton, PhD, a research scientist, cell biologist, and former professor at the University of Wisconsin Medical School and Stanford Medical School. In his book "*The Biology of Belief*", I found a confirmation, an "evidence-based" support to my notion that we are more than our biology. Ideas and perceptions sometimes have the force of a hurricane, and the idea that beliefs control biology was one of them. To learn that we are not at the mercy of our genes and that what we learn and believe becomes hardwired in our brain was a life-changing discovery. To realize that these hardwired programs command physiological responses to environmental challenges was just the cherry on top. Now I know that environmental influences like stress, emotions, and nutrition—not genes—are what determine our blueprints for living and surviving. (Lipton 2005)

My wife and I have researched cancer for almost thirty years, acquiring in the process valuable information that became the base of my therapeutic approach.

The purpose of this book is to describe and to discuss what we learned in these multiple roles: as a patient suffering from cancer, as a caregiver supporting and motivating a spouse diagnosed with the sickness, and as a practicing psycho-oncologist working with clients diagnosed with cancer.

This book is not about fighting cancer. It is about living with the sickness, controlling it, and reducing it to a minimal expression. It is about life, health, beliefs, and hope—which are the most important ingredients in a prescription for happiness and of a balanced life. It is about the people I've met and worked with while teaching, learning, and practicing my craft; and it is about the learning I've obtained through dialogue with my clients while searching for solutions to problems we encounter in the process of living and accommodating ourselves to our changing circumstances and, most importantly, about the problem-solving capabilities exhibited by my clients and non/clients while living and accommodating themselves to these circumstances. It is also about living in fullness; about rediscovering and utilizing the biological, cultural, and psychological tools we possess to attain wellness; and about confronting sicknesses with the tools we are endowed with by nature, such as immune system protection, resilience, creativity, and imagination—adding into this equation emotions, feelings, hope, and spirituality.

This book is also about dealing with the fear that the husband/wife/companion experiences when his/her life partner is diagnosed with cancer. When dealing with the sickness, fear is a big obstacle; for it blocks determination and hope. While fulfilling our role as caregivers, our body language must transmit strength and determination because our energy and attitude will motivate our partner to become fully immersed in the quest for the recovery of health and healing.

The guiding purpose behind writing about these experiences is to convey to you my belief that, in order to attain health, we have to access the information connected to the sickness that is contained in the state-dependent memory and learning of the client (or unconscious mind if you prefer it). In order to achieve this connection, my tool of choice is the use of hypnotic techniques—the creation of a trance state that will allow me to peruse this information.

The second guiding purpose is to put forth the idea that there are clinical and transpersonal ways to help biomedicine to solve the problem of ill health.

Arnold Mindell, PhD, made this second reason explicit by stating that medicine's central job is supporting awareness of the subtle forces of life through a mixture of biomedicine, traditions, and physics—something he calls Rainbow Medicine (Mindell 2004, p. 13).

The most compelling personal reason that motivates me to walk into a territory that is still not well accepted by many practitioners, scientists, and lay people is to research pathological experiences influencing emotional balance; the way by which these pathological sets compromise the effectiveness of our immune system, and how instrumental a trance state could become in bringing back the efficiency and adaptive capability of this system to attain health and healing.

Dr. Hans Selye mentioned, while dealing with his own cancer problem, that he was a scientist; and that "the relationship between stress and cancer is rather complicated," (Siegel 1998, p. 71). Evidence based science is of the opinion that if a phenomenon cannot be subjected to measure, the resulting information does not qualify as science. Unfortunately for science, there are many things that are not measurable: hope, compassion, kindness, determination, fear, negativism, love, enthusiasm, resilience, discouragement, curiosity, etc.

Many of these feelings become strong motivators for a person to direct his inquisitive mind toward the discovery of things. I believe that, before a scientist takes the decision to dedicate his life to science, there is a compelling emotion pushing him toward research to prove to himself and to others his scientific belief. A discovery is not a coincidence. Prior to a discovery, an overwhelming curiosity (you cannot measure curiosity) compelled this researcher to look for the detail, for the tiny Batesonian difference that makes a difference.

In my area of interest, this difference is hope and resilience—both elements present in each one of the cases wherein, against all odds, healing took place. Some people call these situations "spontaneous remission." I call them the result of the combination of resilience, meaning, hope, and science. It was the combination of three of these factors that, between 1973 and 1976—during the Pinochet Military coup orchestrated against the democratically elected government of Salvador Allende, and in the Argentinean military coup orchestrated by Videla against the government of Isabel Peron—allowed me and many others to survive imprisonment and torture in several concentration camps and secret torture chambers.

But this is another story waiting to be written.

In this work, I will be combining personal experiences with supporting scientific information. I beg the reader to be kind when I tend to digress into something academic, for this is the universe I am coming from; and it is quite difficult to shake it off. The other reason for becoming a bit academic is because I want to convey to my readers that this is a road already walked on by many, but most of these people did not write about it.

Since I am a transpersonal/integral therapist, I tend to favor the use of the transpersonal model of consciousness; for it incorporates the perspective of traditional schools of psychology with science, beliefs, spirituality, and dreaming. In the world of transpersonal psychology, perspective, relationships, intentions, and beliefs are more important than tools and methods. Moreover, both my client and I are connected by our personal experiences. Neither is right, wrong, correct, incorrect, healthy, or unhealthy; for our experiences provide only information devoid of personal judgment or personal bias.

Another important transpersonal tenet is the notion that what we believe is real.

Essentially reality is not what it is but what is perceived.

Reality, therefore, is a very personal opinion always subject to change.

I choose to work with non-ordinary states of consciousness because they give me access to the vast domain of the unconscious, to the state-bound experiences we all unconsciously accumulate while living and experiencing the world. These experiences include the perinatal domain; for I believe that by the time we are born, we are already in possession of the intrauterine experience, recorded as state-dependent memory and learning in our unconscious mind.

Since the mind-brain cannot "*not*" learn, we normally accumulate a vast amount of information through our visual, auditory, kinesthetic, olfactory, and gustatory sensory channels; and all of this information, independent of individual volition, are unconsciously accumulated in the mind-brain as a state-dependent memory and learning. This information, which is out of the reach of consciousness, creates opportunities for unwanted behaviors and somatic manifestations that are at the base of immunodeficiency sicknesses, including the proliferation of cancer cells.

The benefit involved in working with non-ordinary states is that I can access these unconscious sets through channels already researched in their effectiveness. One of these channels is Dr. Herbert Benson's Relaxation Response, which allows access through meditation to the state-dependent contents of the mind via the creation of a light trance state. Trancework is another tool to access state-bound information at an even deeper level. Trance is, in Rossi's opinion, "one vivid example of the fundamental nature of all phenomenological experience known as state bound" (Rossi 1986, p. 41).

My clinical experience in the south of Chile taught me that it is feasible to manipulate immunomodulation in people suffering from cancer. Moreover, it taught me about the difference in outcome between those clients that assumed personal responsibility for their treatment and those who delegated their healing responsibility in practitioners (nurses, MDs, clinicians, etc.).

Those clients who assumed personal responsibility in the management of their sickness experienced a faster recovery from ill health than those who were passive recipients of treatment. The first ones felt empowered by the opportunity to work on their own recovery, whereas the second ones suffered the consequence of having no control or role in their own healing process.

Every history of success that I researched indicated the strong presence of "the human factor"—somebody, an individual, a physician, or a practitioner that made a difference in a client's life.

Every story—of the many I've read and/or experienced while doing my clinical work—taught me that drugs, surgery, or radiation alone did not solve the problem. It was this human factor, this resource within or outside the client, the element that motivated him to actively participate and assume responsibility in his healing and recovery.

In my clinical work, I battled with the semantic difference between the concepts of *recovery and healing*. While recovery is more of a physically based change, healing is more of an encompassing process that involves the body, emotions, beliefs, and behaviors, including in the process the special relationship that is created between the client and the practitioner during treatment. Bernie Siegel, MD calls this relationship "the healing partnership", and in defining this relationship, he cites Albert Schweitzer's statement:

"Medicine is not only a science but also the art of letting our own individuality interact with the individuality of the patient." (Siegel 1998, p. 33)

Another finding was the semantic difference between sickness and illness. While illness is conceptualized as the physical or psychiatric symptom or damage visible to a practitioner, sickness is the patient's subjective experience of the disease. Ken Wilber adds that in any disease, a person is confronted with two different entities: (1) The actual disease itself—a broken bone, cancer, or diabetes—is called "illness", which is value-free (no true or false, good or bad).

(2) The way a society or a culture deals with illness—such as judgments, fears, hope, myths, stories, values, meaning, and emotions experienced by the client—is what we conceptualize as "sickness." (Wilber 1998, p. 42)

An interesting aspect of my clinical experience was the opportunity I had of working with clients from the Mapuche

Nation in Chile, as well as with clients from the Cree First Nation in Canada. In both cases, I had to adapt my procedures to their particular healing spirituality, which added valuable learning to my professional background. These experiences will be analysed in a separate chapter.

In order to illustrate some concepts, I am drawing ideas and information from my clinical experiences with some of my clients, as well as from experiences that belong to the public domain.

For the purpose of protecting my clients' privacy, their names have been changed.

THE RESILIENCE FACTOR

First meetings are very important. Our clients are coming to see us when a physical and emotional pain they cannot control possesses them. They are in distress; therefore, we need to give them right away something that will ameliorate their pain and induce hope. They need to understand their past experiences, work in the here-and-now, and project their life toward the future. Time is of the essence during the first interview because we need to bring them back into homeostasis, into a state of personal balance.

My primary goal is to create a hopeful scenario, as well as to help them to become aware that they have within the confines of their bodymind the tools to solve their problem.

When we meet for the first time, I spend a great deal of time conversing with them about resilience and meaning. I explain in detail that all of us are endowed with the most fantastic set of tools to adapt and to survive in any stressful situation no matter how tragic or traumatic this event might be. I also explain that through resilience, we can achieve an emotional and physical balance to counter the often unknown stress created by this out-of-ordinary circumstance we call sickness. Resilience is a normal tool in our tool crib, which is used unconsciously to cope with new situations. Most importantly, living involves a continuous process of adaptation to new situations.

In this initial stage, I apply a principle that I learned, curiously, while being held prisoner of conscience during the military regimes of Pinochet in Chile and Videla in Argentina between 1973 and 1976.

"No matter how desperate the situation might seem, I am here in the present. And this present—which involves everything I am, I possess, I am suffering with—*it is still a resource*, for it has to have something positive in it. My role is to find these resources and use them to build the platform from which I am taking off into the future."

This is the reason why I do not commiserate with my clients. Commiserating will block their creativeness and will regress them back to the situation they were experiencing prior to deciding to come to consult with me.

Storytelling is a great tool to convey ideas and to illustrate the notion of resilience and meaning.

I usually start with stories of common families from the Araucania, which is the place where I was born, guiding my client toward becoming the storyteller of his/her own stories wherein resilience was a factor. Invariably, they discover that there are valuable episodes in their lives that demonstrate that, at one point in their lives, they were resilient heroes.

These stories help the client to shift frames of perceptual and cognitive reference (Lankton and Lankton 1983, p. 66) and reorganize information at the unconscious level.

These are some of the stories I share with my clients to create basic, elemental awareness about resilience and meaning.

Story One

There was this couple living in a small town in the southern part of Chile. They had thirteen children. All of them survived out of love and an uncanny knowledge of the goods that the land was providing. In each season, they went out to collect goods from the wild. The children collected Cuie Colorado (Red Cuie or Culle), a plant with a small red flower—which the mother cooked and reduced to red flat, very sour tarts to be used in winter as cold and flu remedies. Along with these herbs, they collected coguiles, quilo, copihue fruit, dandelion plants, mastuerzo, berros (watercress), and placa to be consumed as salads. In spring they collected Peumos, Gargales, and Changles (Chinese mushrooms). In summer they collected Chupones and Maqui. A wild plant named Yuyo was collected to replace spinach's and Swiss chard's nutritional properties.

People from their community were accustomed to seeing them go on their expeditions to the wild and search for wild berries, fruits, and wild salads to supplement their diet. It was very difficult for a railroad laborer to keep such a large family educated, fed, and alive without relying on what the land offered to them for free. The father died on September 6, 1995, at approximately 103 years old, out of the first sickness that took him to a hospital—a bowel obstruction that required an operation. The mother died in February 10, 2009, at the age of 101 years. Three older children also died: one at age 60, in a domestic accident; and two of cancer, at age 76 and 80. The rest of them are still alive. They are still strong and healthy. Most of them are professionals and highly motivated individuals exhibiting in their quest for higher education the same resilience learned from their parents.

Story Two

There was this child—the son of a maid, a single mother that came from the rural area to work in town. This child became a remarkable student. He was always smiling and happy, growing under the close supervision of his mother. Every summer he walked all over town to tutor his classmates for free, always happy to help. During his years in high school, he endured discrimination from a teacher that made special efforts to highlight the fact that he was the love child, the illegitimate child, of her father.

He is now a mining engineer, still a people's person, loving and loved by his family and peers.

Francisco O. Valenzuela Ph.D.

Story Three

There was this young child that came from the rural outskirts to the same town. He was a child that pushed aside every obstacle, like finances and distance, to become what he is today: a mathematician emeritus of a prestigious university in the United Kingdom, knighted by the Queen of England for his contribution to the space program, adding in March 2012 a Doctor Honoris Causa awarded by the Universidad de la Frontera in Temuco, Chile, one of the universities where he taught prior to being expelled from Chile, in September 1973 by the military regime.

These and many other cases illustrate the power of a resilient spirit to overcome difficult situations. These people's upbringings were quite hard, but their lives had a purpose—the same purpose, the same resilience, and the same spirit that I had to nurture in clients facing life-threatening illnesses. The other connection with these histories has to do with the problem-solving capabilities exhibited by these families and these individuals when confronted with obstacles. I am of the opinion that a sickness is just another obstacle to overcome. It is no different than hunger or poverty. It is a problem that has the same characteristics of any problem. We have to confront it; we have to control the fear and stress generated by the problem; and we have to solve it with all the physical, mental, and spiritual tools we were born with or acquired along the road.

Solutions to physical, emotional, and psychological problems do not entirely come from outside sources (such as health practitioners or our local pharmacy). Most of the solutions come from within, from the self-healing mechanisms we are born with; therefore, *healing is the product of meaning and empowerment.*

When a catastrophic sickness happens, we first open the door to incredulity, physical and spiritual pain, fear, hopelessness, and lack of control. This is what is generally called entropy, which is a lack of order or predictability or a gradual decline into disorder. We then face the dilemma to either succumb to the sickness or to fight it with all our physical, mental, and emotional resources. The same resilience we use to rebuild a house, a life, a financial situation, or a family can also be instrumental in rebuilding our health. It is a personal decision, and all of us are capable and qualified to take it.

Ill health is just another of the many problems of adaptation we face every second; every problem-solving principle is therefore applicable to this situation.

As you can see, the principle that lies behind this writing is a very simple one. It even has a short name: self-empowerment.

Additionally, my client is my main source of information and is my specialist on himself; therefore he must be positioned as a bona fide member of the healing team, with equal participation in treatment planning and decision-making. After all, it is *"the client's"* health and *"the client's"* bodymind we are dealing with.

Moreover, I am of the opinion that when a practitioner wants to explain a concept (such as emotional and physical pain, fear, or anger), the practitioner should feel free to examine his or her own sets of personal experiences and select the ones that are closely linked to the concept he or she is attempting to teach.

Teaching from experience has an amazingly convincing power.

I learned that experiences are perceived through a very idiosyncratic prism. As per Steven Covey's statement, perception and acceptance of an experience as a personal phenomenon make this perception credible and honest. A person cannot act with integrity outside of his perception. This is the real value of personal experiences. (Covey 1982, p. 5)

My own life journey has taught me that the value of past experiences lies not in its classification as bad or good but in the learning we extract from them.

My clinical approach relies primarily on the patient's transpersonal dimension beyond the cognitive-behavioral domain. This dimension includes feelings, emotions, beliefs, socio-cultural environment, and especially the patient's subconscious or unconscious resources and experiences.

While working with altered states of consciousness,[1] I discovered that in every situation in which healing happened, the patient seemed to forget how sick he was. This amnesia-like phenomenon seems to be a powerful defense mechanism that the mind-body possesses to separate from a negative and/or painful event. Because of this, if the practitioner is looking for recognition for a work done well, he will find to his surprise that the client will not remember that he was very sick and that the practitioner was instrumental in his recovery; therefore, not much recognition will come to this committed clinician.

Because I am working with physicians, nurses, and personnel attached to medical clinics, I am using the notion "client" and "patient" indistinctly to refer to the person we are working with.

I like the concept of "client" because it is more dynamic than "patient."

"Client" implies a dialogical level and a participating relationship, whereas "patient" implies a passive and not-so-participating or egalitarian relationship.

Finally I would like to briefly introduce the reader to the definition of Psycho-oncology, the science behind the concepts I am discussing in this book.

> "Psycho-oncology is defined as the sub-specialty of Oncology dealing with two psychological dimensions: (1) The psychological reactions of patients with cancer and their families at all stages of disease and the stresses on staff; and (2) the psychological, social, and behavioral factors that contribute to cancer cause and survival . . . (as well as) . . . concerns for survivors and their psychosocial issues". (Holland et al. 2010, p. 10)

---

[1] An altered state of consciousness is any modification of awareness, including daydreaming and sleep, or any state in which perceptions are different than normal (author's note).

PART I

THE VALUE OF EXPERIENTIAL LEARNING.

Therapeutic Trance and Psycho-Oncology
Using Trance in a Clinical Setting

In March 1997, I began working part-time as a clinician at the Pain Clinic in the Temuco Regional Hospital in Chile. It was an opportunity to work with the most vulnerable population of the Araucania: the Mapuche nation, the urban unemployed, and the needy. It was an opportunity to test the accuracy of the thesis that therapeutic hypnosis can indeed produce changes in our psychobiology and that, by adding trance to communication, we can reach deep into our psychobiological matrix, accessing and modulating mind-body healing resources. In other words, this was an opportunity to demonstrate that hypnosis was not a tool for "feeling good." On the contrary, through anchoring a trance state and solving the riddle of why he became sick, my client and I were able to influence the activity of his immune system (immunomodulation) through accessing the contents of his unconscious mind—contents that are normally beyond the reach of consciousness (his transpersonal domain).

[2]Additionally, Rossi mentions that ideosensory (converting an idea into an act through our visual, auditory, and kinesthetic senses) and ideomotor reflexes convert hypnotic suggestion into body processes (Rossi 1986, pp. 20–21)[3]. This conversion is part of the information transduction in mind-body healing.

Transduction is the basic process of converting or transforming energy or information into psychosomatic expressions or problems.

Basically, unconscious information can produce a sickness in the same way that the manipulation of unconscious information can produce healing.

I believe this dynamic is also at the base of people somaticizing, which is the tendency to experience and communicate emotional distress in the form of physical symptoms.

Adding to Rossi's theories, Timothy Wilson stated, "The mind operates more efficiently by relegating a good deal of high-level, sophisticated thinking to the unconscious" . . . "The adaptive unconscious does an excellent job of sizing up the world, warning people of danger, setting goals, and initiating action in a sophisticated and efficient manner." He added that consciousness is a limited-capacity system and that judgments, feelings, and motives occur outside of awareness. To explain the limited scope of consciousness, he stated that our limited conscious modules couldn't see much of what we want to see. (Wilson 2002, pp. 6–14)

Based on Wilson's findings, my clinical question was: would hypnosis, connected with individual feelings, emotions, and beliefs, be effective in altering the course of immunodeficiency illnesses such as cancer?

The immediate drawback in the hypothesis was the issue of competency. I am aware today—as I was in the past—that there are a number of incompetent people practicing hypnosis without the proper clinical background and, in the process, discrediting one

---

[2]   Therapeutic hypnosis has a long history. In 1886, Bernheim described hypnotic suggestion as a process of "transforming the idea received into an act," i.e. "When I heard about this horror, I became sick to my stomach."

[3]   Ideomotor reflex is a voluntary body movement made in response to a thought or idea.

of the most organic and natural tools for healing and change. Stage hypnotists and I are not very good friends.

Hypnosis and the Trance state have been researched to satiety. There is a 1944 reference to the work of Spiegel and Spiegel[4], which was actualized in 1973.

I agree with them in that hypnosis is not in itself a therapy but a component of treatment.

In my experience, I conceptualize trance and hypnosis as two different entities. While trance is a naturally occurring state common to every human being, hypnosis (or hypnotic manipulation) is a technique and a method for inducing trance to allow an individual to concentrate intensively on a theme.

Trance is involved in every normal cycle occurring to man. Hypnosis is a technique that utilizes normal trance cycles to induce an altered mental state.

In Lawrence Rossi's words, we are like any creature or plant. We are creatures of rhythms and cycles influenced by seasonal rhythms: infradian rhythms (like menstrual cycles), circadian rhythms (like the daily alternation between being awake and asleep), and ultradian rhythms (like the 90- to 120-minute alteration of basic rest). The last one is what I use in trancework.

Trance is everywhere; even professionals that work at the cognitive-behavioral level produce a trance state in their clients because a trance state, like sleeping or breathing, cannot be avoided or suppressed.

Modulating the Immune System: A very important endeavor indeed!

A while ago, while reading Noam Chomsky's dynamic approaches to linguistics[5], it occurred to me that if we

---

[4] Herbert Spiegel, MD and David Spiegel, MD authored one of the first manuals in clinical hypnosis as early as 1944 and revising it in 1978.

[5] Linguistics is the study of language and its structure. Psycholinguistics is the study of the relationship between linguistic behavior and psychological processes (Author's note)

communicate through surface and deep linguistic structures and that if these communications can generate behavior-altering content, we could apply these linguistics modalities (particularly the deep linguistic structures) to alter behaviors of being sick. It could then be possible to connect trance, linguistics, and oncology, subsequently creating a way to alter the behavior of being sick with cancer.

We communicate using surface structures. It is the way we show in the surface what we want other people to know or to understand, but the real communication—the meaningful expression that produces transformation—is connected with the deep linguistic structure. We cannot produce meaningful change unless we work with the structure that is connected to meaning. The surface structure is the face; whereas the deep structure is the heart and soul of the communication, the guardian of meaning and motivation, and the module we have to access to produce remission. In my training in Ericksonian Hypnotherapy, Dr. Milton Erickson insisted that the unconscious mind, containing these deep linguistic structures, normally achieve amazing feats because the unconscious mind is our multitasking system; therefore we should trust its problem-solving capabilities, allowing it to work by providing only general, "artfully vague" commands.

The unconscious domain is conceptualized as the one containing any process of which the personality is unaware but which is a factor in the determination of conscious and bodily phenomena. (Erickson and Rossi, p. 424, as mentioned by Lankton and Lankton, p. 8)

These authors further state that the unconscious is a complex set of associations wherein experiences are automatized. This tends to confirm our inability to control unconscious contents therefore leaving us only with the possibility of "making suggestions" to this wiser module in its use of problem-solving capabilities to—— in the case of sicknesses like cancer—maintain health or affect experiences in a positive way; hence, there is a need to provide the unconscious with a wide set of possibilities so that it can choose the one we want to see happening.

Cancer is a sickness difficult to describe and to treat. Most cancers in adults have been linked to social environment, lifestyle, and psychosocial factors influencing immune function. If psychosocial factors can negatively influence immunomodulation (thus opening the doors to the onset of cancer), the same rationale can be applied to influence immunomodulation to alter the experience of cancer.

The question is . . . how?

While pondering this question, the work of Ernest Lawrence Rossi came again to my mind. Rossi studied the works of the physiologist Hans Selye and of the psychiatrist and hypnotherapist Milton Erickson. He linked Selye's formulation of the General Adaptation Syndrome (GAS) with the concept of state-dependent memory and learning[6], resulting in state-bound information and behavior (Rossi 1986, pp. 57–66). Previously, Selye had followed Walter Canon's concept of "homeostasis," linking his concept of a self-regulating organism with his own construct. Selye stated that, whatever the source of biological stress intruding upon an organism is, it would react with the same pattern of response to restore its internal homeostasis (balance). He further explained that in the GAS (or biological stress syndrome), we could distinguish three stages: (1) the alarm reaction, (2) the stage of resistance, and (3) the stage of exhaustion.

Rossi suggests that the first two stages are connected with his own research in state-dependent memory and learning. The *alarm* reaction is produced via activation of the sympathetic nervous system, which stimulates the release of epinephrine and norepinephrine from the adrenal medullae. These are the same hormones that modulate the retention of memory, making the learning and memory acquired during the alarm reaction to become state-bound and sealed in the unconscious mind.

Selye's second stage, the stage of *resistance*, is the period marked by psychosomatic symptoms becoming evident. The original stressor, which is the drama that I customarily research in my

---

[6] State-dependent or state-bound information is loosely defined as data encoded in our memory (author's note).

5

clientele suffering with cancer, becomes blurry in the effort of the body to "*adapt*" to the new circumstances. The psychosomatic reaction then might become instrumental in the generation of cancer. As per Rossi's statement, "The psychosomatic mode of adaptation was learned during a special (usually traumatic) state-dependent psychophysiological condition. It continues because it remains state-bound or locked into that special psychophysiological condition even after the patient apparently returns to his normal mode of functioning" (Rossi 1986). This would explain the onset of cancer in my wife happening after we were free and living in Canada, which could be construed as a manifestation of the third stage of Dr. Selye's theory: the stage of *exhaustion*. This notion has been confirmed in each and every case of cancer that we have treated in our office.

I am suggesting that, in order to alter the state-bound information and behavior (the behavior of "being sick with cancer") concurrently with the medical treatment, we should endeavor to reach the deep structures of the mind (the unconsciously encoded information of the client's personal tragic experience) and reframe the linguistic structures maintaining the state-bound information (changing the meaning of the tragic experience)[7] by using trance communication as a vehicle to access the neural programs supporting this behavior. Once accessed, we can decode distressing symptoms (taking them apart and reframing them) via suggestions containing general, "artfully vague" directives for alternative behaviors (home work for the client to do after the session). These behaviors will in turn motivate the immune system to collaborate with this change in the same fashion that we hypnotically alter pain nociception.[8]

The role of therapeutic communication (such as the induction and maintenance of trance) is to create a special psychological

---

[7]   This is what Milton Erickson called "inner resynthesis," allowing the unconscious mind to transform the information "unconsciously" (author's note).

[8]   Nociceptors are receptors that can detect and trigger physical responses, like the expression of pain. (Author's note)

state in which the patient can re-associate and reorganize his inner psychological information and utilize his own capacities in a manner according to his experiential life . . . Therapy results from the inner resynthesis of the patient's behavior achieved by the patient himself; it is this experience of re-associating and reorganizing their own experiential life that eventuates in a cure. (Erickson 1948, as mentioned in Rossi 1986)

Moreover, it is the act of indirectly reformulating the deep linguistic structures of the client.

The whole process is, therefore, a communicational event.

Finally, I would like to emphasize that in the process of influencing the immune system, I am clearly staying away from achieving insight. For I believe that the unconscious module of the mind is more powerful and has more tools than our limited conscious module; therefore I carefully follow Milton Erickson's directive to "trust my unconscious mind" and be "artfully vague" in providing commands to our (my client's and my own) unconscious mind. Our unconscious minds will understand and "trance-late" the message in a way so complex that its understanding is beyond the capability of the conscious mind, for the conscious mind does not have the space or capacity to absorb what is unconsciously learned (author's emphasis).

This is basically the difference between Freud's notion of unconscious work and Erickson's notion of unconscious functioning. The first one searches for insight, whereas the second one avoids it.

Using the trance state allows me to communicate with the encrypted content in my client's unconscious mind. This content is rich in experiences and information, for it is the mind's reservoir of knowledge accumulated since childbirth—or in Stanislav Groff's opinion, since inception.

If at any given time we are bombarded by 11 000 000 pieces of information, out of which we can process only forty consciously, my logic tells me that it would be more productive to work on the 10 999 960 bits that are contained in our unconscious mind. (Wilson 2002, p. 24)

7

I would like to mention some of my clinical experiences as a way to illustrate the tenets discussed in this work.

The Case of Elizabeth

Elizabeth, a chartered psychologist, was diagnosed in 1981 with breast cancer. After a partial mastectomy, radiation followed with all its physical and psychological consequences. At the time, I was surprised to discover that there was very little attention placed in the psychological well-being of cancer patients. Ten years later, another cancer followed. She survived both cancers, realizing that what triggered her cancer was connected with her life experience as a victim of the Chilean military coup of 1973 and with the trauma associated with the losses experienced as a Chilean expatriate.

Every research in mind-body medicine indicates that there is a strong connection between trauma and cancer. In her case, September 11, 1973, marked a departure from her and her husband's pleasant life as university professors in the southern part of Chile. A military coup made thousands of Chileans victims of another holocaust. For her husband, this meant concentration camps and torture; for Elizabeth—already pregnant with her youngest son—this meant a hastened departure (to avoid imprisonment) to Peru and later to Argentina.

In Argentina, she started experiencing arthritis and diabetes. When United Nations sent the family to Canada, these symptoms worsened; and finally she became a cancer patient. Her enormous resilience, born out of her resolve to keep on taking care of her family, was a strong motivator for Elizabeth to keep on functioning and to heal.

In spite of all the efforts of the excellent Canadian medical system, an otherwise healthy young woman became a frail and depressed person. Her personal, traumatic experiences seemed to be the tragedy that left her immune system weakened, opening the gates to many immunosuppressive-opportunistic illnesses including cancer. This also explains the high incidence of cancer in males and females in Chile as an after-effect of eighteen years of dictatorship.

Elizabeth is uncommonly gifted in self-modulating her immune system toward recovery. She is currently recovering from yet a third cancer. As of August 2014, she is successfully controlling her third bout with cancer; and all her scans are revealing that this cancer is in retreat.

She has been able to "live with cancer" (as her oncologist posited) since 1981. She is presently a retired psychologist.

Freesia's Case

In 1999, while working with cancer patients at the Pain Clinic attached to the Regional Hospital in Temuco, Chile, I had the privilege of working with Freesia, a staff of a clinic in the Araucania.

A nurse from the pain clinic referred Freesia to my office. She presented a Krukenberg tumor—which was described by the oncologist as a mucocellular carcinoma of the ovary, metastasized from the intestinal tract, characterized by areas of mucoid degeneration and the presence of signet-ring-like cells. The tumor was surgically removed, but the metastasis was well spread since this type of tumor was the result of an advanced gastric carcinoma.

Her prognosis was poor; I was informed that most patients with a Krukenberg tumor die within a year. On February of 1999, she was declared terminally ill with a prognosis of three to five months to live.

When I received Freesia for the first time in my office, her emotions were in disarray. Fear dominated her thoughts. She was a casebook example of a client going through a panic attack related to post-traumatic stress disorder. The use of conscious visualizations at the beginning of the treatment and followed by a deep state of trance were necessary to counterbalance these emotions. Instilling her with hope, conditioning her to a new therapeutic approach she was unfamiliar with, and providing constant education about the functioning and control of her immune system were all necessary to keep her on task in every session.

During the initial interview, her sister explained that Freesia was a widow and the mother of a fifteen-year-old teenager whose only way to cope with her mother's prognosis was to misbehave and do poorly at school.

Freesia was in shock and unable to talk.

The initial interview, in which I attempted to induce a deep trance, lasted for two and a half hours. This was an easy task to accomplish because Freesia utilized the trance as an opportunity to escape from her symptoms. (In similar cases, patients in shock are in a light trance state; therefore, trancework can be applied successfully to deepen this state.) I used glove anesthesia to reduce her abdominal pain. Glove anesthesia is a hypnotically induced absence of sensation in a hand, one that ends at the wrist. During a deep trance, this lack of sensation can be irradiated from the hand to other organs by commanding the client to touch painful zones and to create analgesia in the touched part.

Freesia developed a new sense of trust and hope. Freesia's discovery of her hidden capabilities for symptom control gave her an overwhelming sense of security. For the first time, she felt she could control part of her sickness. And as a consequence, she provided herself with something she was badly in need of: pain relief and hope.

The primary clinical goal was for her to recover her emotional balance and for me to instill hope for healing on a regular basis. It was very important for Freesia to understand and internalize the concept that each one of us carry within our mind-body (bodymind) the cure for any sickness and that healing is within the scope of our immune system. Freesia's assimilation of this information served the purpose to counterbalance the shock produced by the announcement by her oncologist that there was nothing else that he could do for her.

We agreed to work every day for two weeks. After two weeks, we decided to reduce the sessions to twice a week. During most sessions, I used trance to control Freesia's pain and fear. We agreed that if there was a possibility to reverse the course of the disease, she was to immerse herself completely in the treatment.

Freesia's confidence grew with each session, and she perceived herself as feeling better. Her goal was to take control of her body, her emotions, and her sickness.

Freesia and I agreed to team up with members of her family, and she invited her family physician to come to one of the sessions. She not only defeated her fears, but she also extended her life well beyond the five-month initial prognosis. Little by little, her health improved. She walked with the conviction that for as long as she kept focused on recovery, she could achieve control over her sickness. After eight months of treatments, we changed to weekly appointments.

Freesia became a symbol of what a strong resolve and a mind set on healing could achieve. The five-month deadline went and with it her fears. She helped me with other cancer patients, telling them how well she was progressing. Her family physician from the Pitrufquen Hospital was closely monitoring her progress. Even her oncologist from the Temuco Regional Hospital admitted that her cancer was in retreat. Her fears were replaced by a strong confidence in the capabilities of her immune system to eliminate cancerous cells.

On December of 1999, I returned to Canada leaving Freesia under the care of another practitioner. Freesia was apparently unable to develop a healing relationship with her new therapist.

We kept in touch via telephone and e-mail, and I noticed that she felt a void in her treatment. A telling behavior of her loss of confidence was her confession to me; she said that she went to see her oncologist and asked how much remaining time she had. The same professional that initially gave her three to five months to live now gave her an additional two years.

Fear returned.

On June of 2000, I went back to Chile and worked again with Freesia for a solid month. On March of 2002, I received in

Canada the news that she had died exactly two years after her last prognosis.

I have been asking myself what would have happened if we had continued our intense therapy beyond December 1999. This is one question that will remain unanswered.

In spite of this sad outcome, Freesia outlived the Krukenberg prognosis of one year (at the most) for almost two and a half more years.

Freesia's case taught me the damaging effect of fear and hopelessness in lowering the effectiveness of the immune system. She extended her life well beyond any expectation. Even if at the end she succumbed to cancer, her case clearly demonstrated the benefits of a mental, emotional, and physical focus on recovery.

Freesia was a client with an uncommon knowledge of her sickness. She was herself a health practitioner and had readily available help from practitioners from the same hospital in which she was working.

Freesia's case outlines very important points: (a) The patient must become an active participant of the healing team; (b) As much time as needed should be allocated to the treatment; (c) This particular experience demonstrates the value and usefulness of medical hypnosis in the treatment of fear, instillation of hope, and management of cancer pain.

In this particular case, hypnosis as means for pain management and pain control became an effective tool for symptom resolution. Freesia's personal discovery that she possessed the ability to alter her physiological patterns of pain acted as a potent motivator, more so in the presence of an anomaly such as a Krukemberg tumor. In her situation, her ego-strength increased with the newly discovered possibility of her participating actively in her own recovery. Her discovery that she could ameliorate her pain without opiates gave her an insight into the many possibilities available in her bodymind to control her sickness. Moreover, it provided her with an awareness of how instrumental pathological behaviors were in the onset of cancer.

The possibility of achieving something considered impossible gave her strength and hope. The absence of an alternative allowed her to deeply concentrate on healing.

She became a highly motivated client.

One of the most remarkable goals she attained was the control of fear and of panic episodes. She was aware that panicking was dangerous because in the past, panic disabled her problem-solving capabilities.

While under treatment, she felt protected and secured in the notion that she could regain control over her mind-body. In the precise moment in which she felt again vulnerable and insecure, her fears returned with devastating consequences to her health.

From the initial session, Freesia demonstrated to be an excellent hypnotic subject. I spent no more than ten minutes in inducing a deep trance, for she was eager to reach her inner resources. As the case progressed, I could use more precise directives, having no need to be "artfully vague" with the instructions delivered during therapy. We both knew that we first wanted to achieve anesthesia and control of the inflamed tissue. We both wanted this situation to be reversed; we both were concentrating on cancer remission.

As per Erickson's utilization therapy tenets, we utilized every resource Freesia possessed—both physically and psychological—to achieve what she truly, truly wanted, which was healing.

Salvia's Case

On July of 1999, a pain clinic referred Salvia, a forty-one-year old female who was the mother of two young adults, one just graduated from the military academy and the other was a university student.

Salvia's body had developed countless malignant tumors. When one of these tumors seemed to be under control, a metastasis was produced (i.e. a new cancer developed). She had been producing tumors since 1996 when her first melanoma was removed from her forehead. One year later, she developed a malignant breast tumor on her left breast. A radical mastectomy was performed, and a course of chemotherapy was initiated. A while after her breast cancer intervention, it was discovered that some tumors were spreading to her lungs. Metastasis to the liver was investigated, and more courses of chemotherapy were prescribed. Additional tumors were discovered on her thorax. On January of 2005, she had a cyst removed from her thorax; and on December of the same year, a small lump in her right breast was removed. Another one was removed shortly after.

In 1999, the clinical interview revealed the following:

- Right after finishing high school, at age seventeen, Salvia was married to a man who she did not know very well and was fifteen years her senior.
- Her parents decided that she should get married after her older sister became pregnant while single.
- Her father, afraid that the same could happen to Salvia, decided to marry her to a then foreman of a lumberyard that showed interest in her.
- Salvia can be described as a very timid, amiable, and trusting person.
- She stated that her husband never had any meaningful communication with her.

The husband spent most of his time working as an owner/operator of a furniture manufacturing shop, dedicating little time to Salvia and her children.

In Salvia's opinion, her husband perceived his role as one of a provider and that everything in his household should be subjected to his control. He had total control over the family decision-making and finances, having no sharing of responsibilities with Salvia— whose role was reduced to cooking, housekeeping, and child rearing. When she wanted to visit her family, living 250 kilometres from her town, she had to ask permission from her husband and request the necessary money for the trip, which normally consisted of money for the tickets and food. She had no access to any of her husband's bank accounts.

Year after year, her self-esteem deteriorated. She had no permission to work outside of the home or to create her own business. At one point, she was allowed by her husband to open a little craft store in which she used her creativity to fabricate and sell her own creations and other goods. As soon as her business became successful, her husband decided to close it alleging that two businesses were not to his advantage. Immediately after, Salvia started feeling physically sick. In 1996, a melanoma in her forehead was discovered and surgically eliminated.

My work with Salvia consisted mainly of emotional support, empowerment, and reframing of experiences. She perceived her life as devoid of satisfaction. After her mastectomy, she felt the rejection of her husband toward her body. He refused to physically touch her again when she lost her hair.

It is axiomatic that when we develop an illness of the magnitude of cancer, we need the support of family and friends. Salvia's emotional needs increased every time another tumor showed up. Every time that a new growth was discovered, her husband reacted with anger and frustration; and he blamed her for her perceived inability to regain health, obviously having no understanding of her illness. He seemed annoyed by his inability to have control over this situation. He also refused to participate in a support group that would provide him with some understanding of his wife's illness. There was also the issue of financing her treatment. It demanded extra money being spent on trips, lodging, medicines, and medical services—expenses that he resented.

Denial, grief, anger, and depression were present early in Salvia's life. She and her husband were unable to connect on how to deal with her sickness and its aftermath.

It took many sessions for Salvia to look into her feelings toward her body being mutilated and feeling no longer feminine or desirable to her husband. She spent many days at her daughter's apartment, trying to regain her self-confidence. She concentrated on her role as a mother and took care of her daughter's needs.

As a result, mother and daughter created a strong sense of interdependence, almost a symbiotic relationship born out of their desperation and common need for protection. An important motivation for Salvia to survive was her realization that should she die, her daughter would be neglected in her needs—especially where her studies were concerned. She stated that she knew that, to her husband, his daughter's pursuit of a professional designation was a waste of money and time. This belief was confirmed in a telephone conversation in which her husband stated to me that he did not need a university degree to succeed in the furniture manufacturing industry and that women should marry and have children.

My job was reduced mainly to reframe the negative and pathological messages left by Salvia's husband, as well as to reinforce her ego strength. It was an uphill effort wherein only her daughter was a bona fide ally.

On November of 2008, I received news that Salvia had died of a heart failure while receiving chemotherapy. In spite of living in a very toxic family environment, her resolve kept herself alive for twelve years after her first cancer was discovered.

Meaning as a Therapeutic Tool

Viktor Frankl, in referring to Freud's etiological beliefs, stated: . . ."

> It is not possible to cope with the ills and ailments of an age such as ours, one of meaninglessness, depersonalization and dehumanization, unless the human dimension, the dimension of human phenomena, is included in the concept of man that indispensably underlies every sort of psychotherapy, be it on the conscious or unconscious level". (Frankl 1978, p. 13)

It is this human dimension which encompasses all the patient's emotions and feelings, the element that makes the difference between sickness and health.

Since physical health cannot exist in the absence of emotional health, the therapist pursues this human dimension to extract and utilize all the resources available within the patient. Following Frankl's statement, that meaning has an obvious survival value. We can state that resilience and hope are the by-products of meaning.

A hopeful person is a resilient person capable of overcoming every obstacle that life places in his/her path. In a way, Viktor Frankl became significant in what relates to my understanding of resilience and personal beliefs—as well as a motivator in my process of adjusting to a new society, in the realignment of my life, and in the clarification of life goals. We both suffered the loss of our lifestyle, families, groups of reference, language, and freedom. We both witnessed the destruction of lives at a tragic scale, the loss of freedom, and the confinement in concentration camps; and when we realized that we survived this barbaric holocaust, we were faced with the same task to reaccommodate ourselves to a new life, new language, and new customs and to confront our losses with the philosophy that our time to mourn had to be included in the process to reaccommodate and to thrive in a new world.

Similarly, hope and resilience were the elements that kept us physically healthy while interned in concentration camps during the Pinochet regime in Chile and the Dirty War in Argentina. Our minds were concentrated in every feasible way to survive and to keep our mental sanity. During that time, each of us had the perception of ourselves being politically, ethically, and ideologically correct while also assuming that this event was a logical response in opposing our just cause. We conceived that the regime was fearful of an impending turn of events. These beliefs kept us physically healthy; no one in my group suffered even a cold spell in spite of having to sleep on the floor with no covers other than our own jackets and the odd blanket. Our experience corroborated the fact that fatalistic and self-defeating thoughts were the product of the inability to find meaning and a sense of purpose in our existence.

We were well aware that there was a meaning in our physical and mental suffering.

For several years we waited and kept hopeful that a change was going to happen at any time. Our ideals of a just society made us think that this was simply a hiccup in the development of a more humane society. We were still useful for our cause. We had to show that in spite of our condition of oppression, we were neither afraid nor repentant of our principles. In spite of being deprived of our physical freedom, we had a purpose in staying alive.

The same occurred to my wife, who perceived her role as of a person using her freedom to keep the name of her husband in front of the international human rights organizations that were keeping track of people who were in prison or who had disappeared. Her search and keeping our children protected were her main purpose. I neglected to mention that at that time, she was pregnant with our youngest child.

During this period (1973–1974), she maintained perfect physical health. When everything was apparently over, and we were living in Buenos Aires, Argentina (1974–1976), she started showing the first symptoms of her sicknesses. Her bodymind finally acknowledged the pressure she experienced during her search. Unfortunately, we did not have the opportunity to attend to her health: a new military coup—this time in Argentina (1976)— forced her to resume her search, for I was again imprisoned by the Argentinean army who, following the instructions of the "Operation Condor" (a policy of extermination of expatriated by the Chilean, Argentinean, Uruguayan, and Paraguayan armies), zeroed in on Chilean and other South American expats living in Argentina.

After a while, under the protection of the UN, we were expelled from Argentina and sent to Canada.

Salvia's Meaning of Life

In Chile, Salvia was struggling for meaning. She sought shelter in any person that was close to her. She even spent many days at her daughter's student residence in search for a protected space and for a role that could reinforce her struggle for survival. She wanted to live, but the protection she sought was elusive. I noticed that she used her space with nurses and physicians to create an emotional barrier, a cocoon of sorts to protect her childlike self, while fighting with depression. Searching alone and without direction was a terrifying experience, and fear was hindering her capacity to establish a will to live. In this case, individual therapy was a must because the forces that victimized her seemed to be stronger than her resolve to keep her role as a mother and protector of her daughter as a sole reason to survive.

At the beginning of her ordeal, she started writing her experiences, thoughts, and feelings in her private journal. Unfortunately, her husband found and read her diary and physically punished her because he did not like her diary's contents.

Should she decided to abandon this abusive marriage, the Chilean laws were not yet equipped to protect her physically and financially; and she was not emotionally or physically capable of taking care of herself. This situation worried me as a therapist—especially because her husband, due to religious reasons, despised clinical support for her wife.

I felt powerless in front of her tragedy. I felt her passing as one of my professional and personal failures.

A Faulty Meaning?

While researching how meaning affects the life we choose to live, I came across a thesis submitted as publication to the college of Graduate Studies and Research in partial fulfillment of the requirements for the Degree of Master of Education, in the Department of Educational Psychology of the University of Saskatoon, Saskatchewan, Canada. It is titled "*A Matter of Life and*

Death: A Phenomenological Journey". The author chronicled her own death and dying journey. Notable is the purpose of this research, which is the study of the life-death interface utilizing two sources of data: free-associative journal accounts, and dream accounts and their interpretations.

Throughout this particular research, the possibility of surviving is conspicuously absent, almost as if surviving would have hindered the achievement of the purpose of the thesis.

Data collection started in March 1992 when the author realized that her cancer had metastasized to her liver. She apparently programmed herself to die right after the thesis was defended. The epilogue states . . . "(Name erased) defended this thesis on December 09, 1994. On February 18, 1995, (name erased) died peacefully surrounded by her loved ones."

What sets this document apart is the fact that meaning, as well as her hopes were concentrated on having the time to finish the study to attain her Master of Education degree. In researching the background of the applicant, there was a total absence of biographical information, family structure, and dynamics of inter- and intra-familial relationship that could shed some light on the author's life prior to the onset of the sickness. I interviewed the person that gave me the copy of the published research. Apparently, there were a myriad of tragic events that corroborated a simple fact: cancer, in most cases, flourishes in the presence of uncontrollable stress.

This thesis is available to the public at the library of the University of Saskatoon, Saskatchewan, Canada.

Based on the analysis of the aforementioned cases, we can conclude that mind activity elicits physical responses. In the case of health and healing, these physical responses supported by deep-rooted individual beliefs are what Dr. Benson calls the "faith factor."

If perceptions create physical responses, symptoms are the result of conscious and unconscious perceptions.

Our thoughts trigger chemical reactions in our body that are beyond our control. Every infinitesimal mental construct produces a physical reaction which, connected to a set of thoughts, generates a behavior that can be negative or positive.

Conscious and unconscious thoughts develop into conscious and unconscious actions that subsequently produce a state of health or sickness.

The social and emotional environment within which we live will elicit congruent physical reactions. Our lifestyle, our stress level, our happiness (or the lack of it) will influence our mental and physical health.

In my opinion, meaning is behind any story of success or failure. A meaningless life connects us to failure and sickness. Conversely, a meaningful life is behind any story of success and healing. Viktor Frankl stated:"

Man is always reaching out for meaning; in other words, what I call the will to meaning is even to be regarded as man's primary concern . . ."(Frankl 1984, p. 31)

A Cancer-prone Country

Uncontrolled fear and uncertainty are two powerful emotions that can destabilize not only the individual bodymind, but also the whole society, generating massive health problems that might not be perceived as a collective problem by the public health authorities.

Such is the case of Chile and its people.

After the Chilean army military coup of 1973, the "Vicaria de la Solidaridad", an organization created by the Catholic Church to protect the lives and well-being of people being persecuted or imprisoned, published a document titled "*Trauma, Bereavement, and Healing*" (writer's translation from the original "*Trauma, Duelo y Reparacion*) in which a team of mental health practitioners chronicled some of the cases they were attending to. They stopped short of giving the whole country a psychiatric diagnostic. Stress and the unpredictable stability of the nation gave birth to a whole generation suffering from the effects of this enormous social and political disaster. The sense of personal and family safety was erased; and for many years, the whole country lived under curfew and military rule, in which life depended on the whim of the lowest ranked soldier. Many crimes were committed with total impunity, and the life of every inhabitant was out of balance. The only constant was the enormous fear generated by this repressive government's dictatorial rule.

The document of the "Vicaria de la Solidaridad" describes the initial reactions of the people to the news of confinement, death, or disappearance of loved ones. Reactions ranged from one of pain, horror, a sensation of a catastrophe happening in front of their own eyes, incredulity, confusion, and impotence to a quiet resignation. The first reactions were shock and a deep emotional imbalance produced by the irreparable loss, anguish, suffering, and emptiness that seemed worse than the worst nightmare; then they were followed by the inability to accept such an unjust and senseless loss. (Vicaria de la Solidaridad 1987)

Catastrophic illnesses flourished under this regime. The individual's physical and emotional balance was lost. Clearly the mind-body could not adapt to this stress.

Even today, with a democratically elected government in place, there are people that are still experiencing nightmares and ill health as an aftermath of the events that happened in 1973.

In Chile, as of 1990, cancer was the second cause of death in individuals above the age of five. Each year 400 to 480 new cases of cancer appear in youngsters under fifteen years old. In the Araucania Region of Chile (where I practised and is also the poorest area of the country), there were thirty new cancer cases per year in children under fifteen.

In the year 2000, 25 percent of deaths were due to cancer.

In general, mortality due to cancer has constantly increased; and during the last thirty-five years (which coincides with the most tumultuous years in the Chilean history), the male mortality increased dramatically, especially in individuals over sixty-five years old. Chile has one of the highest mortalities in the world due to gastric cancer with the highest indexes happening in Region IX, the Araucania. (CONILE 2003)

On February 03, 2005, the semi-official newspaper, *La Nacion*, mentioned a study produced by Italian researchers, published in *The Annals of Oncology*, and edited by the Oncology Society of Europe. This study concluded that Chile, together with Argentina, have the highest rates of mortality due to cancer in Latin America. The researchers analyzed the patterns of mortality during the period of 1970–2000, which encompassed the most turbulent years of both countries—with the Dirty War in Argentina, in which countless of opponents of the military regime either disappeared or were assassinated, and the military coup in Chile, which followed the same pattern of the Argentinean nation.

Notable were the comments of some mental health organizations that, in 2008, were wondering if the most recent outbreak of consultations to mental health practitioners was connected to the recent court sentencing of the most important members of the secret services of the Pinochet era. Apparently, the people were revisiting that historical period due to the Valech Commission's disclosure of the atrocities committed by the Chilean armed forces. (Valech Commission 2004)

The Chilean experience created a dramatic opportunity for the body to react unconsciously against a psychological injury

I am aware that there are many stories of success and failure of treatments, but the intention of this work is to provide some experiential impression connected with cases in which there has been a degree of success that can be duplicated in the work with other clients. Furthermore, I am of the opinion that cancer cannot be treated in brief medical sessions. Instead, we have to complement the physician's care through working with the client's transpersonal dimension; we have to work inside of the patient's mind, soul, and spirit, consequently making this endeavor require a personal commitment from both the clinician and the client as a condition to achieve success.

This treatment modality requires a flexible and personalized approach tailored to the patient's unique circumstances. The emphasis must be placed in positioning the patient as the main actor of the healing process, with the clear goal of achieving self-healing. Moreover, I am convinced that the problem is not a sine qua non element to the solution; for the problem, manifested as disease, might be misleading. Whatever our unconscious mind thinks, it is manifested in behaviors that in turn translate into physical problems. The real problem lies in the way the unconscious mind is programmed for success or failure.

Our bodymind acts upon these programs and makes real what we are mentally rehearsing.

Based on this principle, I posit that the connection between unconscious motivations and the immune system is the main vehicle in the maintenance and recovery of health; every medical and psychological effort should be directed toward reinforcing its capabilities.

We already know that fear is behind entropy, an inevitable and utter deterioration of the physical and mental balance of our very own systems—our immune system included. Every effort must be directed toward restoration of balance (homeostasis), which is the necessary balance that the client has to achieve in the sickness–health equation. Moreover, it is important for the practitioner to recognize that the main source of information is the patient himself, who should be listened to with profound respect and attention. After all, he is the mind-body unit we are working with; and he knows more than we do about his symptoms and feelings.

In my practice, I realized that trancework is instrumental in the recovery of the client's personal balance through constant unconscious monitoring of the client's allostatic charge. "Allostasis is the capacity to adapt or constantly change through modifying physiological and behavioral parameters in order to adjust to ever shifting environmental conditions." (Fricchione, G. 2011)

PART II

EMOTIONS AND HEALTH

"Happy people do not get cancer, unless they happily smoke themselves to death." (A nurse at an Aboriginal Clinic in Northern Alberta)

This statement may hold some truth after all. My experience with cancer patients taught me that behind every adult cancer patient, there is a tragedy to be uncovered. Not long ago, a physician from InspireHealth (an organization in British Columbia, Canada, who supports and provides integral medical services to cancer clients) said to me that the role of the practitioner is to maintain our cancer cells dormant for as long as possible. One of the important processes to keep them dormant and to neutralize their activity is the monitoring of emotional states.

Pain and suffering, though normal to every individual, could dramatically affect the functioning of the immune system. Doctors Hans Selye and Herbert Benson already demonstrated that anxiety and chronic stress inhibit the immune system thus reducing resistance to sickness. Blocking negative emotions without resolving them decreases even further the capabilities of the immune system to fend off disease.

Gregory Fricchione, MD, states that this is a manifestation of *allostatic loading*, which is the physiological consequence of chronic exposure to repeated or chronic stress. It is the wear and tear the body experiences due to constant exposure to suffering. Anxiety and depression are allostatic load disorders. (Fricchione 2011)

Suffering

Deepak Chopra is an excellent author that goes beyond the physician's procrustean bed. In connection with the September 11 attack on the world trade center towers, he talks on the matter of suffering. He suggests that suffering is the pain that makes life seem meaningless. He adds that humans are subjected to complex inner pains that include fear, guilt, shame, grief, rage, and hopelessness. (Chopra 2002, p. 31)

He distinguished three stages of suffering that are common to any tragic situation. Taking this even further, I am of the opinion that these stages are basically the same for anybody suffering a catastrophic illness.

The first stage consists of experiences of numbness and shock.

Shock gives way to tears and grief. Safety is thought on the most basic levels; and the individual seeks shelter within, concealing even his most basic emotions, thus allowing no one to share in their pain. Our client turns himself inward.

It is the "why me" stage.

Even in the New Testament, Jesus, being the Son of God, expressed his fear and desperation in his saying "My God, my God, why hast thou forsaken me?"

I know about intense fear through personal experiences, and I am aware that many physical and emotional reactions take place in an instant. I am also aware that under duress, we tend to doubt our capabilities to fend off disease and survive the ordeal.

I do not have to navigate any further from my own experience as the spouse of a cancer patient, remembering (almost thirty years after) how I tried to numb my mind out of my wife's diagnosis of breast cancer.

On October 15, 2010, a good friend of ours was diagnosed in the worst way by an uncaring physician who told her in my presence . . . "There is nothing that I can do because inside of you, everything is terrible . . . terrible! There will be no surgeon that would touch you, and you might have three months if you are lucky." After witnessing this physician's action, I had to go home, embrace my wife, and ask her for forgiveness for my lack of sensitivity years ago. I felt guilty—even after thirty years—for not being as supportive and as sensitive as I should have been. If I had known then what I know today, I would have surrounded her with all my love. Perhaps I did it, but I am still unable to recall the first month after the diagnosis and of any action that I initiated to ameliorate her pain and fear.

2. Second Stage: Powerful emotions rise to the surface.

The shock connects with pre-existing emotions. Some of these emotions might have been buried for years. Sorrow erupts and fear shows. Any incident triggers panic. Anxiety peaks.

While reading Treya's statement after finding out she had breast cancer in *Grace and Grit: Spirituality in the Life and Death of Treya Wilber*, I did recall our fear mimicking Treya's . . . "*I am shocked, almost frozen. I don't cry. In a dazed kind of calm I ask several intelligent questions, trying to hold on, not daring yet to look at Ken. But when Dr. Richards leaves to call a nurse, then, and only then, I turn to look at Ken, stricken. I burst into tears, everything dissolves around me . . .*" (Wilber 1993, p. 33)

Treya's shock made me remember the horror of facing something that was totally out of our control while listening to the physician explaining that my wife had a malignant tumor in her right breast. I felt a strange feeling of shame associated with what was happening as if we were guilty of this terrible diagnosis . . . shame and guilt associated with my perception of us, my perception of what we became—people separated from their roots because of political, ethical, and philosophical beliefs . . . guilt associated with my own inability to protect her and for involving her in this unplanned journey as Chilean expatriates.

3. Third stage: The sufferer takes action, either toward healing or seeking protection in a quiet state of resignation and despondency.

In this stage, the sufferer examines all the possible alternatives in conscious and unconscious ways. This is the stage in which critically ill patients start looking for any or every possibility to deal with a negative prognosis: fighting or flying, seeking solutions, or simply resigning themselves to mourn their impending death. This is the very moment that forces the practitioner into searching for the most sophisticated tools in his psychological arsenal to reframe the client's perceptions and to position this client toward attaining health.

Dr. Stanislav Grof qualifies these situations as psychological emergencies, suggesting that these are magnificent opportunities to focus the client toward healing through transformation. A critical illness like cancer would qualify as a "spiritual emergency" or a crisis of transformation, a radical personality transformation, and a spiritual opening; it is a psycho-spiritual crisis that can bring about emotional and psychological healing and consciousness evolution. (Grof 2000, p. 137)

It is as if the body finally asks in the worst way for attention.

The common denominator in all of these stages is stress, fear, and anguish.

Fear that is not directed toward a concrete external object or situation becomes anxiety—a nonspecific emotion, something internal happening in response to something vague and hard to identify. It is a subjective state of apprehension and uneasiness, a typical expression of allostatic load.

Like fear, anxiety affects the whole being. Like fear, anxiety produces reactions on physiological, behavioral, and psychological levels.

Are all Emotions Important In The Equation Sickness-Health?

(. . . Thank goodness for old curriculums . . .)

Milton Erickson MD was a master in utilizing natural life experiences, ordeals, and confrontations. He was a creative problem solver, never afraid of using client's personal traits to reframe a state of mind. The following example, in my opinion, follows typical Ericksonian guidelines. (I could never imagine then that this would be a banner case in my professional practice.)

In 1966, I was attending the School of Social Work at the Universidad de Concepcion (University of Concepcion) located in the southern part of Chile. This school prepared social workers to work in remote communities as community developers; therefore, we were to be prepared for almost anything. The school had incorporated in its academic curriculum a twelve-month program of general medicine, which covered from first aid and advanced first aid to introductory gynecology, obstetrics, and basic pathologies. The idea was to create a professional flexible enough to discover and basically diagnose illnesses with potential for propagation to a whole community, as well as being capable—in the absence of proper assistance—to attend somebody delivering a baby, providing at the same time the necessary education to provide proper parenting skills to their parents.

One day, my brother-in-law (then a social sciences teacher) signalled me to approach, confiding me that he had something odd on his testicles. To plain observation, they were swollen and unnatural-looking. Since in the preceding weeks we were studying all sorts of cancer manifestations, I assumed that this looked very much like cancer of the testicles. I told him that it might be cancer. (In this situation, ignorance was a blessing because today I would have not dared to say what I said without taking the person to see someone more competent than I was, such as a physician). He went to the hospital, and in the same day, he was booked for surgery. He was not told very much about his situation. The next day, he was told that his testicles had been removed.

Depression ensued and he started radiation treatment, which made him very ill. At that time, there was no professional support, no psychologist to prepare him emotionally to deal with the disease and to assume his loss.

He prepared himself to die even though through all his life, he had demonstrated an enormous courage to progress and study unaided by parents, siblings, or student's grants or loans. Until his surgery, he was a self-made and resilient individual.

On the days following surgery, all of us searched for some pharmaceutical help as coadjutor to the radiation treatment. The answers given were always like a kiss of death. A pharmacist, after I told her the story and asked her for some miraculous remedy (In Chile, you can obtain all sorts of medications over the counter), commented back to me that she was prepared to help with the orphans and the widow.

To everybody, my brother-in-law was as good as dead. He became bedridden, asking to see his family. In the meantime, I took over some of his classes as a substitute teacher. We needed his salary to survive. After all, I was living in his house while going to the university.

He was bedridden and depressed, and his only sibling came to visit him at his request. This sibling, by his own design, decided to take his brother out of his bedridden, depressive condition by utilizing a very personal shock therapy.

He was uncannily cold and insensitive to my brother-in-law's demand for emotional support. He stated that he was a very busy individual and that he did not have time for dying people—not even for his brother. If he needed money, he could give it to him; but he could provide neither his time nor his emotional support because he had neither time nor energy for either.

My brother-in-law reacted furiously, stating that he was neither sick nor in need of handouts from anybody. He instantly came out of bed; and on the next day, he went back to work, enduring at the same time radiation therapy.

Today, almost fifty years later, he survived a quadruple bypass and is still working in his areas of interest: sociology and education.

His recovery is still a conversational piece at his brother's cabin on the Lake Lanalhue, where their families spend most of their summers. It is a known fact that his brother saved him by using a very natural and organic shock therapy. My brother-in-law's immune system and emotions did the rest.

Is There Any Relationship Between Emotions and Health?

Robert Ader, a psychologist from the University of Rochester, discovered that the immune system is capable of learning in the same fashion the brain does. A biological pathway connects the nervous system and the immune system, creating a unique unit encompassing mind, body, and emotions.

The notion of the immune system as the "body's brain" makes the mechanics of the body's healing processes easier to understand. This discovery has today given birth to a new category of science: Psychoneuroimmunology (PNI).

PNI explains the link between distinct processes that attempt to describe how mental phenomena, such as stress, influences physical responses. PNI encompasses the interaction between mental processes, central nervous system responses, and immune and endocrine functions. The nervous, immune and endocrine systems mutually influence one another. The central nervous system (CNS) influences hormone outputs, and vice versa, different types of hormones act as neurotransmitters. Over and above, the CNS influences immune functioning.

This emerging medical science acknowledges the links between the mind, neuroendocrine system, and the immune system. Moreover, it acknowledges the strong impact that emotions have on the autonomic nervous system, which regulates every function of the body—from blood pressure to insulin production.

The Anger/Stress Factor

Anger has been labeled as one of the emotions that significantly impact the functions of the heart by altering its pumping efficiency, generating myocardial ischemia—a drop in blood flow to the heart. The old notion that depression is a situation of "anger turned against the self" can easily be applied to cancer; for in every one of the cases that I am using as illustration, there is an element of anger present, either covertly or overtly manifested. If anger is connected with depression, and depression with cancer, it has to necessarily be a connection between the psychodynamics of depression and anger and cancer. Once we know about it, we can amplify the opposite notion, using trance to amplify hopefulness and to activate the problem-solving capabilities of the bodymind thus confirming the human capacity to positively modulate the immune system toward health and well-being.

While studying the stress–disease link, Bruce McEwen, a psychologist from Yale, noted that stress effectively compromised immune function—even accelerating the metastasis of cancer by increasing the vulnerability to viral infections, as well as exacerbating plaque formation to generate arteriosclerosis and blood clotting. He also noted the acceleration of the onset of diabetes, type I and type II. The impact of distress in infectious diseases, such as cold, herpes, and flu has already been amply documented. Furthermore, Sheldon Cohen, a faculty member from Carnegie-Mellon University, noted the relationship between stress and the weakening of the immune system. (Journal of American Medical Association 1992)

In my opinion, suppressing anger is as bad as giving to the client a space to "vent" his anger by hitting a pillow or, as a component of therapy, using the therapist as the object of his anger. Suppressing anger demands a great deal of energy, and when this anger can no longer be suppressed, it explodes in the many illnesses the bodymind uses to vent the problem.

Anger is a normal, basic emotion common to every person; therefore, it should be recognized and accepted as something normal. Labeling a natural emotion as bad or attempting to get rid of it is denying its inevitability. Reframing a "negative anger" and transforming it into a "positive anger" is something that Milton Erickson, MD, (probably the most unusual yet effective therapist of our time) would have recommended.

"While we were interned in concentration camps, we learnt to accept the anger generated by this confinement as a by-product or consequence of our political and ethical stance. By accepting this anger, we allowed it to become a normal, acceptable reaction to the real problem, which was the implementation of an authoritarian military coup that destabilized the whole nation." (author's notes)

Stress and the Immune System

Dr. David Felten acknowledged that messages have immune implication, and linguistic utterances can in fact become iatrogenic[9] thus producing iatrogenic sickness or iatrogenic health. Information delivery has a powerful impact on the way our client fights off diseases.

Stress is a fact of life, and it means different things to different people. My accountant in Slave Lake, Alberta, thinks that his life would be meaningless without stress. He stated that stress invigorates him and readies his mind and muscles to spring into action. Conversely, others become immobilized by the fear produced by stress.

Stress-induced anxiety is at the base of many immunodeficient responses to sickness; therefore, stress-coping techniques become a necessity for controlling the symptoms of stress and anxiety.

Balancing the immune system is crucial to maintaining health.

Autoimmune diseases are produced as a consequence of our immune system's defence mechanisms attacking themselves, causing damage and sometimes death. This may be produced due

---

[9]   Iatrogenic. Resulting from the activity of a medical practitioner.

to a special type of cells called regulatory T cells failing to do their job of keeping the immune system in line.

Autoimmune disorders could be caused by viral or bacterial infection, stress and/or genetic susceptibility, which can be studied through biological markers.

In the case of viruses or bacteria, they avoid detection by creating a string of amino acids that mimic those of the body, which are thought of as "self" until an anomaly makes them detectable. The immune system becomes confused and attacks self-tissue. An example of this confusion is the Adenovirus Type-2, which has amino acid strings similar to those of the myelin protein surrounding the nerves of the body. The body attacks the myelin thinking of it as an anomaly.

It is important to remember that immunosuppression, stress, and mind-body connections are intimately related. The perception of distress activates immune messengers and subsequently triggers physiological changes. Fear stimulates the production of corticotrophin-releasing factor by the hypothalamus. This in turn stimulates the release of corticosteroids, in some cases reducing immune system response and decreasing the body's ability to fight off diseases. It is already known that a depressed hypothalamic-pituitary-adrenal axis makes individuals prone to allergies and autoimmune diseases and that the measurement of immune measures (in spite of sounding redundant) is complex. Nutrition and sleep can be measured, but emotions associated with immunosuppression are hard to quantify. In a study about psychological stress associated with susceptibility to upper respiratory infections, Cohen established the existence of substantial evidence that psychological influences play a role in infectious upper respiratory diseases in humans. It is equally evident that psychological stress plays a role in determining susceptibility for some infectious agents. Cohen stated that the magnitude of the effect of conditioning or stress in modulating immune responses of clients depends on the following factors:

- Host factors such as age, sex, genes, or intrinsic immune status
- Quality and quantity of behavioral interventions
- Amount and type of relaxation practices, if required
- Quality and quantity of antigen stimulation or exposure to infectious agents
- Temporal relationship between behavioral and antigenic stimulation
- Nature of the immune response and the methods of measuring it
- Other unknown factors (Cohen 1995, as cited by Themes 1999 p. 35)

Connected to the age factor, I would like to mention that many of my successful clients were over sixty-five years old.

I can safely say today that all of us can influence immune-modulation. We can produce hypnoanesthesia, delaying cutaneous sensitivity. We can increase immune response to antigens, such as cold viruses, and achieve symptom elimination of conditions like allergic reactions to environmental agents such as pollen or dust. In our office, we teach guided immunomodulation to our cancer clientele as part of their training to improve health. Among the most used techniques for immune-modulation are relaxation, imagery, visualization, meditation, and deep trance induction.

Since information and communication are elements that permeate every conscious and unconscious human activity, immunomodulation cannot happen in the absence of a form of communication between a stimulus and the response generated by the mind-body.

We work with symbols and images, and as a result, deep or surface linguistic mental structures are generated by this symbol–image combination. Formal description or mind-generated symbols and images allow the individual to create a mental matrix from which covert and overt behaviors are generated.

Ray Jackendoff, a linguist, describes in his book *Consciousness and the Computational Mind* the many ways in which mental representations are intimately connected with immune-modulation. One of the most salient themes in Jackendoff's work is the modularity of the mind and how it can be further articulated. He states that it is indeed possible to articulate a theory of the central levels of representation of the mind, particularly the level of conceptual structure. This theory states that conceptual structures communicate with each other in the central level of the mind. (Jackendoff 1996)

From a hypnotherapist's point of view, central level of the mind is another name for the unconscious mind, which is capable of connecting all these communications to generate a coherent body of knowledge, which in turn generate an action or behavior.

Whether intentional or unintentional, Jackendoff seems to confirm the basic tenet of Ericksonian hypnotherapy of the independence of the unconscious mind and its capability to re-contextualize problematic processes so they can function as value-able solutions. (Gilligan 1987, p. xiv)

We are still far from learning how to access and utilize these mind-body mechanisms, but even though our knowledge is still sketchy, we know enough to attempt to modulate these systems. So far, the results are promising; for they indicate that we can manipulate unconscious content to create expected outcomes.

Stress and Health

It is quite difficult to talk about stress without mentioning the work of Dr. Hans Selye.

In 1950, Dr. Hans Selye formulated the concept of the General Adaptation Syndrome (GAS). He stated that the internal organs, the endocrine glands, and the nervous system help to adjust to the constant changes that occur in every individual. Failure in this process of adaptation is translated into disease and unhappiness. He further mentioned that man, through the constant interplay between his mental and bodily reactions, has the power to influence this adaptation to a considerable extent. Even if we cannot avoid stress, we have the mechanism to reduce its effect.

Disease is perceived as an outcome of errors in the process of adaptation to stress; many nervous and emotional problems, high blood pressure, ulcers, rheumatoid arthritis, allergic cardiovascular, and renal diseases are diseases of adaptation.

Dr. Selye created the notion of stress to explain that the fight-or-flight response not only as a physiological response, but also as a psychological response of the bodymind to threats. Mental perceptions or worries trigger the fight-or-flight response.

Selye's work allowed researchers to determine that stress and reactions to stress are paramount in the occurrence of health and disease. He also established the existence of good and bad stress. Good stress positions us into "the zone," creating conditions or opportunities for "peak performance." In a way, it is a form of "controlled" stress. Stress over and above what is needed for peak performance (also called beneficial or adaptive stress) becomes harmful, or simply, "bad stress."

Dr. Selye introduced the notion of a Stress-Induced Psychosomatic Symptomatology as well as the GAS, which he conceptualized as the capacity of the mindbody to adapt to stressful experiences. These notions are closely connected with Cannon's concept of homeostasis, which suggests that the body maintains stability and continues carrying on vital functions in spite of dangerous conditions existing in the external environment and internally within the body.

In many ways, the components of the GAS—which are alarm, reaction, and exhaustion—explain why sicknesses like cancer occur in the last stage of adaptability, wherein personal tragedy seems to be over.

While studying Dr. Selye's theories, I came across Bernie Siegel's relation of exceptional patients and of Dr. Selye's experience and ulterior exceptional reaction as a sufferer of reticulum cell sarcoma. I see in this story a close resemblance with the previously told experience of my brother-in-law's cancer occurrence.

This is Bernie Siegel's relation:

> At age sixty-five, Hans Selye developed reticulum cell sarcoma, a type of cancer whose cure rate is extremely low. This is perhaps the ultimate stress, but in an interview, Selye discussed how he reacted to it in an exceptional way. "I was sure I was going to die, so I said to myself, 'All right now, this is about the very worst thing that could happen to you, but there are two ways you can handle this. Either you can go around feeling like a miserable candidate on death row and whimper away a year, or else you can try to squeeze as much from life now as you can.' I chose the latter because I'm a fighter, and cancer provided me with the biggest fight of my life. I took it as a natural experiment that pushed me to the ultimate test whether I was right or wrong. Then a strange thing happened. A year went by, then two, then three, and look what happened. It turned out that I was the fortunate exception!"

> "Afterward I made a particular effort to cut down my stress level. I have to be very careful what I say here because I am a scientist, and no statistics now exist to say whether stress is related to cancer. Apart from the genetic and environmental causes of cancer, I can only say that the relationship between stress and cancer is rather complicated. In just the same way that electricity can both cause and prevent heat, depending on how things are balanced, stress can both initiate and prevent illness."

> (The interviewer asked) "Some people have described cancer as a disease that is somewhat like the body's

way of rejecting itself. Now to carry that premise one step further, could it be that when the people drastically reject their basic needs, they are possibly more apt to develop cancer? In other words, if a person rejects his own needs, can his body rebel and reject itself?"

"I don't say yes and I don't say no. I'm a scientist, not a philosopher. All I can say as a scientist is that the great majority of physical illnesses have in part some psychosomatic origin." (Siegel 1998, p. 71)

In 1950, Dr. Selye could not firmly determine the cause of his cancer, even though he cautiously mentioned that it could be psychosomatic. Nowadays this caution is hardly needed. As per Pasteur's expression, now we know that it is not the seed but the type of soil that one uses that can produce a proper harvest. Pasteur was referring to whether it was the microbe that caused the illness or it was a body that was prepared to accept and suffer with the microbe.

There are other extreme examples of the connection between cancer and stress. The one that I most vividly recall is the work of the mental health practitioners from the Vicaria de la Solidaridad in Chile. These practitioners were dealing with their clients' fears as well as their own since all of them were exposed to the rage and irrational repression of the Pinochet regime. (Weinstein 1987, pp.109–122)

My experience with fear, while a prisoner in several concentration camps in Chile and in Argentina during the repression from 1973 to 1976, allowed me to learn how difficult it is to detach from fear and to observe it from the outside. When I finally managed to learn this procedure, I became an observer of everybody else's behavior while dealing with their personal fears and my own. There were the ones that succumbed to their fear, becoming emotional and behavioral casualties and later (if surviving) becoming long-term clients of the mental health system. The ones with a clear idea of why they were there—the ones politically and emotionally prepared for a possible outcome of suffering and persecution from the regime—were the ones that came out ready to reinitiate a different kind of life, to survive, and to heal. By detaching and observing the phenomenon as outsiders, we were able to prepare and desensitize other prisoners for the incoming experience of torture. We fed ourselves with the hope that a country with a long democratic tradition, such as ours, could not accept a regime of repression and torture.

At that time, we did not know that this state of affairs was going to last eighteen years.

In Chile, about eighty percent of the patients I worked with were women. They were very courageous; in several cases, I saw them walking into the clinic unaided, alone, sometimes with friends, and very seldom accompanied by their husbands. I initially attributed this absence to the need of the husbands to work while their wives were coming for treatment.

I offered to work on Saturdays and on evenings to facilitate their attendance for them to become members of the healing team. They found many excuses not to attend.

I learned that the fear to acknowledge the sickness of their wives was stronger than their need to understand that they were supposed to be part of the healing process. Denial was a difficult feeling to deal with; in several cases, the sickness was attributed to a voluntary inability of the patient to recover.

As of today, it is still difficult to incorporate the family into the circle of treatment. The main culprit is the fear of the unknown and the member's own perception of uselessness regarding what to do hence the need to educate the family for them to understand that they play an important role in the patient's healing process.

Every relative, spouse, or child of a person suffering a catastrophic illness is familiar with the experience of fear that wakes the person up in the middle of the night, bringing this suffering individual to his/her knees. They feel powerless in front of a situation perceived as hopeless, wherein it is difficult to comprehend why this nightmare is happening. Many run away from the situation into a detached and apparently uncaring behavior thus compounding the family tragedy.

The onset of a disability later in life creates havoc in families, forcing dramatic changes in the way they live and feel. A long-term sickness can lead into feelings of being alone, compounded by the enormous financial losses created by the interruption of gainful employment. The individual feels that his body is his enemy, an entity that carries inside something malignant and out of control and allows no space for hope.

How do we neutralize in our head this pathological perception? Is there a way out of this unbearable stress?

These were the questions I was confronted with when I was told that my wife had a large malignant tumor on her right breast.

After dealing with the fear of her impending death, we both realized that we could not simply give in and wait. We had a child that was a toddler and a family to maintain abroad in a country where the main source of income was money sent by expatriates like us to feed the families left behind.

We understood in that precise moment that our lives had only present and future, that the baggage of the past should not hinder the future. We took the decision to work in the present, in the here-and-now, and thereafter projecting ourselves toward the future with a single thought in mind: we could not be defeated by a sickness because many lives depended on our health and earnings.

After many years of keeping her cancer in check, she is still fearful of the day when she has to go for her yearly check-up at the cancer clinic. Year after year, the answer is still the same: she is still cancer free, but the trauma produced by the diagnostic is still permeating many moments of our life.

Projecting us toward the future by working in the present was lifesaving. Today we use the same approach with our clientele. Time is too precious to be spent in the past. If the unconscious mind is our most intelligent part and also our information bank, I can trust that the unconscious mind already knows what the problem is.

As a therapist and caregiver, I just needed to trust my wife's information bank as well as her abilities to reframe her state-bound experiences. Historically she has been able to "transcend and include" most of her state-dependent memories and learning connected with our experience in Chile during the military regime, as well as reframing, transcending, and including the experience of processing and resolving three cancers. These lessons are what she is presently applying in our work with clients that have been diagnosed with the sickness.

The Structure of Fear

Fear is one of the most difficult emotions to overcome. Fear is behind poor relationships, failure, and sickness. Fear leads to hopelessness, dulls our senses, and (once it is internalized and accepted by the unconscious mind) leads us to panic. A sense of doom follows, and the immune system becomes blocked.

From here onward, we are sitting ducks to sickness.

Fear is an omnipresent feeling. We feel afraid of the past, present, future, old age, poverty, and physical and emotional pain. Cancer, in particular, produces a very distinct type of fear which can affect even people that are not cancer patients. It is called cancerophobia or carcinophobia or simply fear of cancer. It is conceptualized as a persistent, abnormal, and irrational fear of the sickness (cancer). This phobia causes panic episodes expressed in shortness of breath, rapid breathing, irregular heartbeat, sweating, nausea, and an overall feeling of dread, fear, and pain. Even though there are drugs to ameliorate symptoms, these drugs do not solve the problems; they just mask them.

Cancer fear, like any phobia, is produced in our unconscious mind by our protective mechanism. It is produced as a response to an emotional trauma linked with cancer. Our unconscious mind classifies the event as dangerous and creates an anchor that triggers the response in every situation that seems connected with the trauma. Fear is triggered by any signal that may indicate impending harm and readies the body for action, which is translated into the fight-or-flight behavior. Like any specie, our protective mechanism has the role of preserving itself.

I remember one of the last comments I received from a friend, a Chilean expatriate physician. He stated that the reason why many women in Chile became pregnant after the military coup was because in nature, species under threat attempt to fight extermination by increasing their reproductive capabilities. To me it was hard to understand that in a situation of danger and instability, when every day and every night we were expecting the secret police to come and seize us, we became pregnant. Prior to the military coup, as young professors enjoying stable and promising careers, we tried unsuccessfully to have a child, not knowing that history was going to deliver us a blow without precedent. The idea of a military coup in our country was simply preposterous. Yet it happened.

It was right after being freed from the first of many imprisonments that we did, in fact, conceive our child.

Was the fear of being exterminated the one that created in us a successful urge to reproduce?

Fear is a complex phenomenon encompassing many emotions. I cried in anger when I realized the betrayal of some of my co-workers and some of my political friends who became informants of the de facto government—some of them even becoming torturers. We adapted to the fear of being caught and tortured or murdered. It was so unbearable that at one point, it did not matter anymore. It was as if a veil of indifference made us oblivious to danger.

Even though I was aware that we are born with an essential fear, and that this fear serves the purpose of keeping us aware of any threat, I could not imagine the extent to which fear could paralyze me to the extreme that I could not even think of a quick way out.

Like children learning about danger, my fear grew spontaneously with the first incarceration and electrical "treatment" (the military called this treatment my "lesson on how to play electric guitar"). With the second and third imprisonment and subsequent "electric guitar lessons," I learned to modulate my fear and change it into *their fear of my payback time.*

I was shocked to read, thirty years later, that this was nothing other than the application of the experiment # 18 of Peer Administering Shocks, devised by Stanley Milgram, who researched procedures on how to facilitate submission to the new authority (Milgram 1974, p. 121). This finding requires a parallel research that is not in the scope of this work, even though it relates to an historical slice of life that presently affects myriads of people in Chile and in Argentina.

Healing requires courage. Fear, on the other hand, blocks any possibility for healing and recovery. Healing differs depending on which stage of anxiety a person is in and how they relate to this fear.

To deal with the emotions of fear, I use distracting comments, knowing that every distraction adds more irrelevant information to the original fear program. During the process of eliciting a therapeutic trance state, I insert topics interspersed with the topic of fear, little by little reframing this experience and transforming it into something completely different. My tools of choice to induce amnesia to the fear are non sequiturs, which are irrelevant topics that are interspersed in the current situation being presented by the client. Non sequiturs create sudden confusion, preventing and altering cognitive processing of the experience. Sooner or later you will find yourself wondering about forgetting to remember about going into a trance . . . (and) wondering how wonderful it would be to think about the thoughts that were not there . . . on a different level . . . (and) about freeing yourself of these thoughts . . . and you may do so suddenly or gradually (a double bind) . . .

These techniques will be examined in a separate chapter.

Because I am certain that one of the most damaging emotions experienced by cancer patients is fear, I attempt in my clinical work to reverse this emotion by creating in my client a trance-state and by providing directives to reframe and transform his fear into a more manageable feeling. Trance can effectively block fear networks, transforming them into a less threatening experience.

Frightened patients are already in an altered state of consciousness; therefore, trance can be induced with ease. While experiencing fear, their understanding is childlike and literal (Rossi and Cheek, 1988); therefore, they are highly vulnerable to harmful suggestions but also highly sensitive to trance inductions.

There are many emotions interacting within the patient's psyche, like guilt, shame, self-punishment, self-loathing, and self-defeating feelings. The critically ill adult also faces childlike fears and night terrors. These emotions cannot be ignored, for they become obstacles to healing.

My connection with these fears comes from a very personal source.

My father was hospitalized for the first time in his life at age 103. Like many men from rural communities, his mind was clear; and his life span was longer than many of the people of his generation. His health was remarkable, and until the day that an intestinal occlusion made necessary a surgical intervention, his health and mind were remarkably functional. After the procedure, he was left unattended in a recovery room. When he woke up, he was disoriented and did not know what was happening to him. He saw tubes protruding from his body and, in a big panic, instinctively took them off. He died one month later as a consequence of this action.

It was indeed, a criminal act of negligence in the care of the elderly, which in many medical circles is considered a waste of time and resources. (Author's note)

I know that disorientation and fear are very common among people undergoing surgery with general anesthesia. If they have little or no experience with this type of procedure, they become vulnerable to potentially lethal panic. This is similarly true for people undergoing chemotherapy or radiation therapy—both of which are very invasive procedures that tend to create havoc among patients because of their highly intrusive nature and potential for producing extensive damage in the patient's bodies, compounded by side effects such as loss of hair, upset stomachs, and deep burns.

To Palliate or not to Palliate: That's the Question!

I am of the opinion that palliative care is sometimes used prematurely.

The World Health Organization defines palliative care as "the active total care of a patient whose disease is not responding to curative treatment . . . The goal of palliative care is the achievement of the best possible quality of life for patients and their families." (World Health Organization 1990)

Palliative care is loosely conceptualized as an interdisciplinary therapeutic model that focuses on the comprehensive management of the physical, psychological, social, and spiritual needs of patients suffering from progressive incurable diseases and their families.

The synonyms of palliate are: to extenuate, to gloss (over), prettify, sugar-coat, varnish, veneer, white, whiten, whitewash, to conceal, to reduce the violence of, to moderate the intensity (Webster New College Dictionary 1976, p. 825). To palliate, in my opinion, tends to eliminate healing and recovery as a possibility by stunting a fighting spirit and decreasing its combativeness. Somehow it translates as accepting a bad prognosis and maintaining the mind-body in suspense while preparing oneself for the worst.

I am not denying that palliative care is an important part of the process. On the contrary, I know that, given certain circumstances, it would be the only help that we could provide to our clientele.

I suggest that before attempting to deliver palliative treatment, we should identify and utilize all the elements that the client possesses for self-healing while empowering him with the belief that he/she has a role in prolonging his/her life expectancy or experiencing remission. When all these attempts fail, we should resort to palliative care.

Since we are already aware of the existence and importance of emotions in the fight for health, we owe it to the client to work toward recovery until it is obvious that the client's systems (or the clients themselves), are not responding to any form of intervention.

As per definition, palliative interventions are geared to maintain the quality of life or attenuate the suffering of the patient and the family. Listed below are some of the assumptions in the definition that merit some reflections.

• Disease is not responding to curative treatment.

Were all the modalities of "curative treatment" considered in this statement? Was the holistic alternative or integrative medicine approach explored, or was only the traditional allopathic, biomedical approach considered? Were all healing approaches already exhausted? Was the singular experience of the patient and/ or his wishes and hopes examined? Who is determining that the patient is not responding?

My experience tells me that sometimes the client surrenders to the sickness as a way to escape from an uncaring and indifferent practitioner. On occasion, this affirmation comes from a frustrated practitioner who failed to establish a proper rapport; and the client was therefore found to be not very responsive or cooperative, or as somebody at a clinic in Northern Alberta put it very bluntly, "If somebody wanna go, we should not concern ourselves with his or her will!" This person apparently did not know about the way a depressed and scared patient behaves.

Many clients that survived cancer did so by exploring other avenues, after traditional allopathic medicine gave up and classified them as "not responding to curative treatment." In my opinion, these "other avenues" should be considered complementary to treatment, not as an alternative to treatment.

• The patient has a progressive incurable illness.

Can we say nowadays that cancer cannot be stopped?

If we ask Lance Armstrong—with a testicular cancer that metastasised to his brain and lungs—perhaps he would have told us that his physician stated that he had a progressive incurable cancer, but in Lance Armstrong's mind, his cancer did not meet this standard.

Several of my clients can testify that there is no such thing as progressive incurable cancer, for in their experience, they have already proved that it is up to their immune system and emotions to determine whether this cancer will progress or stop.

Moreover, the notion of palliative care seems to be absent in the works of physicians like Simonton or Chopra. In my opinion, this absence is not a coincidence because these physicians, like many others, strongly believe in the capabilities of the bodymind to bounce back from even the worst situations.

A very kind physician from InspireHealth (a Vancouver-based cancer clinic) suggested that the role of the practitioner and the patient, united in a treatment process, is to keep the cancer cells dormant for as long as possible.

I still believe that in many hospices all over the world, there are people who could have reversed their illnesses but were never given the chance to do so.

Communicating with the Client/Patient

There is an element conspicuously absent in the illness–healing equation. This missing element is the right of the patient and his family to know and to be informed about any departure from health. An informed person is capable of taking informed decisions and, as a consequence, engaging in an extra effort to save his own life.

Normally a hyper-aroused patient can read not only the physician's body language, but also the body language of anybody that is connected with him. Keeping the patient ignorant of his delicate state makes things worse. In most cases, the client perceives that something terrible is happening; but he does not know the details.

We generally tend to underestimate the capabilities of the clients to comprehend the medical and psychological details of his state. When the client does not know what is happening, his imagination creates a monstrous picture of his state; and his visualizations are many times worse than reality. The imagination leaves no space for hope.

When cancer struck my wife, nobody volunteered an explanation. There was only the urgency to act and eliminate the tumor in her breast. Perhaps it was the right thing to do, but the physician never volunteered much information. We did not know what to do or where to go to get information. We were left with no roles to fill in her treatment.

Cancer meant death, and nobody told us otherwise. We were two blind, scared persons following not-so-clear instructions and, worst of all, having the impression that nobody knew anything or cared about it. We were sent from one place to another, in each place spending hours in waiting, terrified. This was followed by no more than ten minutes of examination by a physician who was acting as if my wife was no different from a broken chair or table. Apparently, she did not deserve explanations; or he felt we were too dumb to know the difference. The only thing we knew was that something had gone terribly wrong. We felt powerless as we listened to the physician telling us that something was there. The mammography did not explain it, but the physician's clinical experience said that there was a tumor to remove and, with it, the whole breast. It was like talking about somebody else, not my spouse. No second opinion, no alternatives. The shock, the urgency, and the lack of explanation about what was happening left us stranded in a process that we did not understand.

Fortunately, there was a physician approaching retirement at the Cross Cancer Institute in Edmonton that gave us her time and kindness to explain, in plain English, what was happening and what the possible outcomes were. It was a long and unusual meeting that instilled hope and decreased our fears to a manageable intensity.

This initial experience taught me that the missing element in the disease–treatment equation is the emotional and psychological support that allows the client to keep his humanity, dignity, and hope intact. These unmet needs increase the emotional fear and loss of control experienced by every cancer patient receiving treatment, leaving them exposed to further immunosuppressive consequences. Many new concepts were learned while listening to the language of this medical environment wherein we had no experience.

Similar to the concept of illness versus sickness, it seems that there was little awareness about the difference in the meaning of concepts like information and experience.

Information is what is exchanged between the client and the clinician. It is concise and value- neutral. It is more or less biographical and statistical.

Experience is the emotional load that it is included within the communication: body language, description of ongoing feelings and emotions (e.g., fear, despair, hope) as experienced by both the client and the clinician. Unlike pure information, experience is exchanged between client and clinician during treatment; for the sharing of experience is an important element in the act of communicating toward healing. This is why handouts are not a replacement for verbal communication, but they should rather be used as support for the verbal communication.

In order to create an effective therapeutic communication, the clinician should observe the problem from the perspective of the client. Positioning the client in the same level would produce mutual understanding, for communication is based on the acknowledgement of both the client's and the clinician's perspective. (Stiefel 2006, p. 2)

A very capable integral coach, Laura Divine, explained that we perceive the client in two ways simultaneously: The first is looking *at* the client to discern what set of skills are needed to balance what is present and what is lacking in the process. The second way is to look *as* the client—which involves being able to look through the client's eyes and to go deep into his mind, body, and soul to get a sense of his unique way of seeing and of relating to their suffering.

In a way, in order to grasp his world, we must "walk in his shoes." Only then will we be able to help this client to "transcend and include" their experience. (Divine 2009, pp. 21–22)[10]

When we ignore the need of the client for emotional support, we eliminate hope and perpetuate fears, with all the added negative consequences.

A sick organ does not represent the person and, by the same token, we cannot treat the organ without treating the whole person. We simply cannot deliver healing in five or ten minutes of treatment. Moreover, healing cannot be the responsibility of only one professional (the physician). This professional normally has a waiting room full of people expecting him/her to deliver time and services.

Healing is the responsibility of a whole milieu; Nurses, therapists, family members, and community support systems must be engaged as members of the healing team. The team's main goal should be the creation of an environment that would allow the client to return to a state of physical and emotional balance.

In order for the client to counterbalance the damage of the sickness—physical, emotional, or otherwise—it is important to convey to this client proper and honest information and feedback.

Inadequate communication exposes the client to a renewed and unnecessary fear. Sometimes this feeling is so pervasive that it does not allow the space for the patient (client) to develop a proper mindset for healing.

To avoid this problem, I would like to suggest the following:

- Each person, with the exception of young children and intellectually challenged individuals, is capable to understand and comprehend the medical details of their sickness.

---

[10] Transcend and Include is a process in which we reach a higher level of knowledge and experience "including" the information obtained in the level we just transcended. (Author's note).

- A proper explanation must consider the person as a valuable human being capable of making his or her own decisions.
- We must avoid creating feelings within the client that they are been patronized.
- In the same fashion that statistical information is provided, we should allow the client access to experiential information about successful cases.
- Hope cannot be overriden by the fear of being hopeful. There is no such thing as "false hope."

I am familiar with the difficulties involved in the creation of meaningful change, but I am also familiar with the difference that meaningful change produces when we provide messages of hope and healing to counteract the effect of a physician's announcement that a case is in metastasis. For many professionals, it is still difficult to accept that our immune system is listening to our mind talk.

The following case is illustrative of the need and value of the creation of an integrative approach as well as a proper communication in a therapeutic setting. I am treating it as a separate chapter because of its uniqueness and because it involves the distinct characteristics of First Nations' spirituality and healing practices.

First Nations' Healing and Spirituality: The Use of Therapeutic Metaphors and Trance States

Case example: Louise

On July 2001, while practicing in Northern Alberta, Canada, I was blessed with the opportunity to work with a client from the area. This experience involved an elderly lady from the Cree Nation, who was suffering from cancer.

The family physician referred Louise to me with the request to deliver some form of palliative care because the laboratory information, as well as his professional experience, told him that Louise was in the last stage of cancer; but this client thought otherwise.

Since the beginning of treatment for a colorectal cancer metastasized to her bones, she had the mindset to heal. In order to reinforce this mindset, I added to the equation the request for everybody around her to join in the same belief. With these two elements under control, we concentrated on healing and recovery.

At the time of initiation of treatment, she was seventy-three years old. As of January 2006, she was still surviving.

This case demonstrates the value of empowerment. When a client acquires the firm, conscious–unconscious cognition that she is in control of her mind-body unit, this client becomes empowered to achieve almost anything, even defeating a bad prognosis. It further demonstrates that the client possesses, beyond awareness, an awesome set of tools for wellness.

One of First Nation's spiritual beliefs is that healing is connected with nature and that sickness is the result of a lack of balance between the individual and his natural and spiritual habitat. Entering a native habitat has to be done with total respect and acceptance of their values. A most important factor in healing is the establishment of an integral patient–client relationship in a unique spiritual connection with nature.

When I was introduced to Louise, she was in a wheelchair, hopeless and depressed. She had a colorectal cancer metastasized to the bones and had fractures in her pelvic and hip bones.

Her nurse informed me that she was receiving opiates for pain and that her moods were swinging due to her pain and her inability to move around to do house chores.

Her prognosis was bleak.

Louise's husband was also disabled as he was suffering from Chronic Obstructive Pulmonary Disease (COPD). A housekeeper was hired from the community to cook and to keep their environment dust-free.

In our first interview, Louise stated that her inability to do house chores depressed her immensely and that she resented her dependence on her housekeeper. Her family was continuously visiting and providing her with emotional support while at the same time asking for resignation and patience, which in Louise's perceptions was an indication that recovery was not going to be attained. One of her children was constantly encouraging her to do the prescribed exercises and to take her medicine. And in order to motivate her to move around, he had carved her a cane to do short walks out of the wheelchair. He was the only hopeful person in the household.

I immediately enrolled him to be part of our healing team.

At the time of my intervention, there were two "terminally ill" cancer patients in that clinic; and only Louise was interested in working with me. I was informed that the other patient, a thirty-two-year-old mother of two, did have family support and was herself a fighter. She was apparently content with the amount of support she was receiving; therefore, the head nurse decided that we should concentrate on Louise's treatment.

I had to explain to the head nurse, and indirectly to the whole staff of the clinic, that my intervention had the general purpose of uncovering the intervening factors—such as pathological and depressive thoughts, feelings, emotions, beliefs, and behaviors—that might have influenced the onset of cancer and that my other purpose was to identify the activities the patient could do to help herself to recover physically and emotionally. I further explained that my interventions were over and above her medical treatment.

I asked Louise for a written permission to talk to her physician, from whom I received a great deal of help. This physician was aware of the benefits of psychological support and had in the past participated in professional development meetings in which the Simonton approach, a mind-body approach to healing in cancer, was discussed. Once I secured Louise's consent, this physician agreed to allow me access to the information in her file and was instrumental in providing and explaining exams such as X-rays, blood work, and laboratory results. The physician and I agreed in the use of an interdisciplinary approach to support Louise's endeavour toward recovery.

The first meeting was dedicated to discuss with Louise the idea that mind and body are interconnected in the same way that man and nature are interconnected and that emotions have an important role in the creation of illnesses, as well as in the recovery from them.

The second idea discussed was that as individuals, we participate in the onset and recovery of our sicknesses and that we are mostly not aware of our participation in either state because most of this process occurs beyond awareness. I explained that in the many cases that I read or were involved in as a therapist, prior to the onset of a sickness, there were tragic or negative events that weakened the patient's immune system. She commented that her life was pretty much an ordinary and uneventful life.

We decided to talk and explore her "ordinary life" to see if we could find some events that could have any connection with her present ill health.

We discovered that there were many unresolved tragic elements in her life: physical and emotional abuse, her life away from her family in residential children's schools belonging to the Catholic Church, the death of her first husband due to alcohol abuse, a child committing suicide, another dying in a car accident, and the sickness of her present husband.

I invited Louise to reflect on these events as generators of negative and damaging emotions, as well as obstacles in stabilizing her immune system. Issues of the past were connected with drinking and physical and mental abuse.

Several sessions were dedicated to talking about these years.

Since the sessions were taking place at their residence, I worked with both husband and wife, each one sitting in a wheelchair, while we were sipping laboom tea, Muskeg tea, or Labador tea (this is how it phonetically sounded)—which, she explained, are herbs widely consumed by the woodland people. Louise stated that these teas were medicinal cleansing teas that were prescribed by a British Columbian Medicine Man.

At the end of these discovery sessions, I proceeded to ask how important it was for her to have a normal life and how committed she would be to a process to recover her health.

She stated that she realized that her job as a *kookum* (native Cree grandmother) was not over yet and that she was worried about the behavior of one of her favorite grandchildren. She said that if she recovers her good health, she would dedicate her efforts to guide him and to nurture him so he would separate from bad company, from bad friends. She reaffirmed this comment by telling me that the role of the Kookum is to nurture and to guide the grandchildren.

It is important to mention that in the native family structure, the kookum is a central member of the family and has a high degree of power to influence family decisions. This role brings, as a consequence, an enormous responsibility, especially in the communications between parents and children.

I asked Louise about her readiness to start her journey toward health and well-being. She answered that she was ready now.

I took this as a strong signal of a commitment to health; therefore, we proceeded to write a contract for wellness.

I usually ask my clientele to sign a commitment to health and healing in the form of a contract for health as a way to anchor a positive thought. Even though some practitioners are of the opinion that these contracts are ineffective, I like to write a contract as a way to create an emotionally binding ceremony toward health.

After the contract for health was signed, I concentrated on the identification of elements in her belief system that could help me to understand her thought processes. I needed to learn the subtlety of Louise's communication, the values contained in her most distinctive words, and the themes that were important to her—themes that were surfacing in her narrative. I needed to make sure that I was correctly interpreting her statements and that we both were building the same bridge.

To this effect, I decided to use some of Paulo Freire's theories of communication, which helped us to develop a rich and productive dialogical relationship. I focused on two linguistic elements: her Vocabular Universe and her Generative Themes.

Vocabular Universe is the identification of a particular linguistic modality that people use in their communication with the environment in which they live and work. This particular linguistic modality is part of their cultural background and is highly distinctive. (i.e. A welder would have a different vocabular universe than that of a lawyer.)

Generative Themes would be the subject or subjects that are of utmost importance to an individual. These themes are connected with the client's value systems and are encompassing beliefs, principles, and life purpose. Every theme is to be identified and used in the generation of new, reframed themes. I am adding more detailed information in the analysis portion of this particular case.

The following themes (beliefs) were identified:

1. Louise believed in aboriginal medicine and in medicine men.
2. Louise believed in aboriginal herbal medicine to be stronger than pharmaceutical products and that herbal remedies are effective as healing agents, for there is a spiritual content in everything created by nature.
3. Louise believed that there is a strong connection between native people and their native habitat and that this connection goes beyond the simple acceptance of her surroundings. She believed that whatever mankind does affects everything around him and that every creature, animal, vegetable, or mineral is interconnected and therefore affected.
4. Louise believed that the role of a kookum is of utmost importance for the well-being of her family.

Once these themes were researched, I explained the importance of rest and relaxation in the process of attaining health. We talked about pain and the many tools the mind possesses to control, manage, and eliminate pain.

I followed with relaxation and mental imagery twice a week.

In order for her to train her mind to create mental images, conscious sets of visualizations were used with open eyes. Progressive approaches to unconscious, deeper imagery followed until she learned to develop eye closure and deep trances.

In order for her to understand and to accept unconsciously the possibility of recovery, I utilized the following changes in season as healing metaphors:

- *Winter* (sickness), a metaphor depicting our bodies suffering from a low-functioning immune system.
- *Spring*, which follows winter as an expression of initiation of recovery.
- *Summer*, which denotes the strongest push of the immune system to empower itself, to be back into high-functioning mode.
- *Fall*, which suggests the elimination of all dead cells and tissues.
- *Winter again* as a time of healing, relaxation, and conditioning for the body to generate new tissues and heal the bone fractures.
- *And again Spring* to celebrate renewed health.

It is important to clarify the different meanings of winter: as a metaphor for sickness and as a metaphor for healing. Winter will happen again and again, and it must be reframed with different meanings. Winter can be perceived dually: as a dreaded season approaching us and as a time for relaxation, meditation, reflection, and renewal.

During the trance sessions, I utilized the following secondary metaphors:

- *Spring house cleaning*, as a time of taking the garbage to the dump, signifying the discarding of dead tissue

- *A house tool crib*, which is a metaphor for the many capabilities of the immune system and a metaphor for the self-healing competencies of the mind-body
- *Closing the eyes to dream*, to acknowledge that the mind's eye sees a different reality.
- *Body scanning with the mind's eye and harvesting the medicinal herbs to give space for the new ones to grow* (metaphor for healing and recovery)
- *A tenant living in the attic and not paying rent and the eviction of this tenant* as a metaphor for bad feelings and resentment that do nothing to help recovery. The same image was used as a metaphor for the elimination of bad cells and tissues.

In order for Louise to get third-party information, I left behind the book *The Healing Journey* by Carl Simonton and Reid Henson. This book relates the sickness and recovery of Reid Henson from metastasized cancer. I made sure that the material was of easy reading and understanding. Third-party information is left to reinforce the content of the meeting, allowing therapeutic content to remain present in the client's mind and keeping the client on task until the next meeting.

Louise and I constantly examined and modified some programmed goals and planned future events. I purposely avoided mentioning her sickness again unless she wanted to talk about it.

The intention was to create a certainty of a disease-free time in the future.

In order to anchor this intention, we focused on issues and events of her interest that she could plan for the near future—like holidays or activities such as bingo or camping at the lake.

We worked progressively under the assumption that her body was eliminating the bad cells and healing the parts that needed to be repaired. A careful monitoring of her commitment to health was done on an ongoing basis.

Every time the nurse at the clinic informed me that something seemed not to be working, I requested an appointment with the nurse to examine the situation, to course-correct the process, and to make sure that Louise remained involved in the treatment.

One of the outcomes of our many meetings was Louise becoming accustomed to being mindful of her feelings and analyzing them every time she felt out of control. As a result, she managed to learn to detach herself from stress-generating issues. In this detached state, she was able to look at the issues from a safe distance, as if they were somebody else's issues.

It is important to explain that Cree people—and, in general, Canadian First Nation people—very seldom like to explore personal issues, such as emotions and feelings, with a non-native person. I do not know nor have I been able to verify whether they are more open to talk about personal issues within themselves. This was my first stumble in the process to effectively communicate with Louise, and I think she decided to communicate with me because she realized that I was genuinely interested in working with her.

In one occasion while visiting her, I noticed that the curtains for one of her windows were full of small, black spiders. In a panic, I grabbed a magazine from a near table and started hitting the spiders only to realize, after hearing a big laugh coming from Louise and her husband, that they were plastic spiders that their grandchild had placed there; for it was the day after Halloween.

They realized that, like any human being, I did have my own fears.

I had to confess to them that I was fearful of snakes, spiders, and rats.

Louise's physician became instrumental in her recovery, closely monitoring her health. At the time of the initiation of my intervention, she was seeing him twice a week. Periodical X-rays provided information on her fractured pelvis. Her physician noticed that her fractures were mending and her tumors diminishing in size.

In the summer of 2002, after one year of treatment, Louise again enjoyed summer camping, working on her garden, and collecting wild berries. The years 2003 and 2004 were remarkable for her. She was again in charge of her household, baking for her family, canning, doing laundry, and enjoying bingo once a week.

While working in the here-and-now, we concentrated on reinforcing the belief of her being instrumental in the unconscious generation of her sickness as well as in her conscious/unconscious healing and recovery. Louise, her husband, and I celebrated the physician's information regarding her fractures and her tumors.

At the end of 2005, my wife and I moved to Edmonton. One of the most notable among the losses I experienced by moving was the loss of my contact with Louise.

Case Analysis

Throughout this paper, I am mentioning the importance of fear in the progression of a catastrophic illness. The pervading effect of fear is most damaging to the healing process. Fear is omnipresent in each and every situation that involves a cancer client.

In our first interview, Louise silently cried out her fear. Typically, she had surrendered to feelings of hopelessness. Her level of stress was high, and she saw herself progressively deteriorating. Hope was low and fears were high. Even her family was expecting a fatal outcome.

One of the persons in charge of community health stated, "We (aboriginal people) believe that we should not interfere with destiny. When a person feels that her time to go is arriving and she has no hope, we should let her be."

As I mentioned before, utterances along these lines coming from professionals or officers in positions of influence and power acquire a definite iatrogenic[11] effect on the client because it completely disregards the importance and influence of individual emotions and purpose in recovering from ill health. An iatrogenic message of this calibre is paramount to the gestation and progression of a sickness. Upon so much emotional pain and

---

[11]   Something with a negative consequence induced inadvertently by a practitioner (author's note).

suffering, compounded by negative messages, the client reacts somatically; then physical sickness follows.

When I went for the first time to visit her at her home, and when asking for directions, somebody asked me "Are you looking for the lady that is dying from cancer?" Of course, in a small community, everybody knows what is happening in their milieu. Louise was aware of it. She did not attend public functions and stopped going to bingo—which is a very important pastime in aboriginal communities—and everybody assumed that the reason of her absence was her advanced cancer. To herself and to the people in the community, it was almost as if cancer could be transmitted aerobically.

Our challenge was to reverse this perception.

To attain this change, I enlisted the help and cooperation of every member of the family and explained to them the notion of behavioral medicine, the mind-body connection, and the concept of cancer as a stress-produced disease—all of it in a language easy to understand.

I asked everybody to produce positive messages in a very casual way. I suggested that visitors should approach the visit not as a visit to a sick person but as the normal visiting of one relative to another. It was quite difficult to change their beliefs, but they desperately wanted to maintain hope. They embraced the possibility of recovery with much-needed enthusiasm.

In order to create positive beliefs, I concentrated on changing their negative thoughts about cancer. To succeed in this enterprise, I decided to enlist the cooperation of somebody in the community with a degree of social prestige and high credibility; and that was the community head nurse. Additionally, I obtained the cooperation of the patient's physician who fortunately was aware of the importance of emotions in the generation and healing of sicknesses.

With the purpose of obtaining the cooperation of family members, I researched the family's belief system and utilized the beliefs that were connected with the endeavour of providing hope.

To train this client in the use of visualizations and trance states, I had to earn her trust and convince her that I had something to offer. Since we were going to use an approach of which the client had no information, I needed to obtain her permission. This was a very difficult task because natives tend to not trust people from outside the community. In my research on their belief system, I discovered the value they place on dreaming and praying; therefore, I explained to Louise that trance was normally involved in native dreaming and praying and that most of the communications between aboriginal people and nature was through dreaming and trance.

Additionally, I provided Louise with educational information on the variety of functions of the immune system and the way it protects the human body.

During all this exchange, I worked on creating a strong rapport. My goal was to convince her to become a member of the healing team. Once this goal was achieved, I concentrated on planning a practical and understandable mind-body model of recovery, congruent with Louise's values and beliefs. The next step was to share this model with her.

I asked Louise to explain to me her role as a kookum. She told me that in this role, she was important and irreplaceable within the family fabric and that, without her assistance, a series of problem situations could become critical.

One of her strongest motivators to succeed was coming from her daughter-in-law. She had a partial mastectomy and was waiting for radiation treatment and chemotherapy.

Louise became her role model.

The reinstatement of Louise's roles as kookum, caregiver, and role model gave her a meaning to live. To Louise, it was of primary importance to provide hope and to influence the functioning of the people she cares for by staying alive and showcasing for them the value of resilience.

It took time, effort, and dedication to create this awareness. The change from a passive patient receiving treatment to one actively participating in her own recovery required a radical transformation of her mental maps.

To achieve an emotional and appropriate connection, I had to research her distinctive patterns of communication. Since communication involves some form of education, Paulo Freire's consciousness-raising method became a most effective tool to educate and be educated by Louise on what it meant to be a Cree person. Traditional allopathic treatment focuses on one person *acting* on another rather than two persons *working with* each other. Paulo Freire's notion of Praxis, which is reflection-action-reflection or value-linked acting, affirms that communication has to be meaningful to make a difference. Communication has to produce a cooperative effort, which must involve mutual respect. This is the reason behind the search for the client's Vocabular Universe, which encompasses all the words commonly used every day by the client, as well as the emotional meanings that are attached to them. This vocabular universe was subsequently used to create the text of the message that I conveyed to Louise's unconscious mind in the forms of directives for healing.

(Writer's note: I was Freire's disciple between 1969 and 1972. The notion is loosely translated from the Spanish and Portuguese *Universo Vocabular* into *Vocabular Universe*. I extracted the word vocabular from the 1976 version of The Webster New Collegiate Dictionary, which defines the word as an adjective: (back-formation fr. Vocabulary); of or relating to words or phraseology; verbal)

Freire researched the vocabulary of social groups during informal encounters with people from diverse communities. This vocabulary was selected based on political or existential relevance or as verbal expressions linked to the idiosyncratic experience of a defined group of people.

The objective of researching this idiosyncratic vocabulary was to create encrypted messages to be conveyed to this client's unconscious mind for it to understand and assimilate valid and useful information, as well as to increase state-dependent memory and information content.

I need to emphasize the understanding that the vocabular universe of a program analyst differs from the vocabular universe of a welder or a lawyer. By using the client's vocabulary and meaningful themes, the dialogue becomes meaningful to this client. This results in a client being consciously and unconsciously informed and also feeling empowered to transform his reality.

(I would suggest the reader to peruse Paulo Freire, 1973, *Education for Critical Consciousness.*)

Finally, I was informed that after we moved to Edmonton, Louise moved to the city with relatives. I could not find information about her whereabouts; therefore, my normal follow up with this client was interrupted.

Louise's Meaning of Life

When I met Louise for the first time at her place, I sensed the sadness expressed in her perceived lack of usefulness as a person. At that time, she stated that she viewed herself as a useless woman, a burden to her family, while suffering from her physical and emotional pains. She was in a wheelchair waiting to die.

The nurse that made the referral perceived my role as simply palliative.

I decided to look for anchors that could give Louise a reason to fight. It was quite a difficult task since she could not find any reason to hope for anything. The only medication she was receiving was opiates.

We had a long conversation in which tragedy cascaded from her narrative. I could sense the stoicism in her stance. The aboriginal strength that kept her alive for over seventy years and the fatalistic perception of her present life as meaningless were constantly present in her narrative.

Based on her story, I conceived my therapeutic intervention as a "meaning-centered therapy."

I could not provide hope without discovering a life purpose. I had in my mind Nietzsche's quote as recited by Frankl: "He who has a *why* to live can bear with almost any *how*."

My mind went back to a conversation with a native lady that I met many years ago while working in a foster parent project in Northern Alberta. She stated at that time that the most important role of a woman in a native community was to take care of the children since they do not belong to just one family but to the whole community. She expounded the encompassing role of a kookum in an extended family system, wherein the kookum is at the center of the family dynamics.

In our first conversation, Louise commented on her despairing inability to attend to her grandchildren's needs. Before she became sick, she was assiduously visited; and she enjoyed entertaining her children with food, sweets, and buns that she baked for the whole family.

I decided to empower the kookum image, and putting aside the medical information received from her physician, I asked her what was the problem and why she could not just continue entertaining her children and grandchildren.

Louise explained that John, her husband, was sick and could not stay in an environment full of dust. She was in a wheelchair because she could not put any weight on her hips since the cancer was already threatening her bones, and she already had some fissures on her pelvis. She felt that these circumstances limited her abilities to fulfill her role as kookum and as a caregiver of her spouse.

It is important to add that Louise stated that she did not receive much information on the particulars of her sickness. What we do not know makes our imagination work overtime. Louise already had the notion that her health was going to be worsening with time.

Louise, John, and I talked about the role of the immune system—that this system was one of her gifts from nature and that it was hers to use. Furthermore, I explained and described the role of the mind in creating images, feelings, and emotions, and that sadness is the prelude to physical sickness. I asked how important children were to her and how her impending death could affect them. She commented that she wanted to be able to again interact with her grandchildren, to entertain them, and to cook and bake bannock for them. Following her comments, I asked her if she would try a different approach if there were a possibility of her recovering because of it.

We wrote the health contract right after she said "Yes!" [12]

We analyzed all the barriers that precluded her from doing what she wanted to do. We talked openly about the future, as if cancer were only a slight inconvenience. In order to achieve her health and family goals, we were going to concentrate our attention in the here and now and in her future.

She decided that she was going to entertain her children again.

We had a meeting with her physician in Slave Lake; and he agreed to join the efforts, providing a very comprehensive logistic support and valuable medical information to help us guide Louise in her quest for recovery. Our primary goal was to have her life purpose permanently in front of her eyes, for her to keep focused on healing.

A secondary goal was to keep her informed about the unique capabilities of her bodymind unit. I wanted Louise to be mindful of her spirituality. I wanted to teach her the ways to master a conscious and unconscious control of her natural defenses. We spent a number of sessions just talking about the many cases wherein people recovered from ill health, and I asked her to tell me about her time in residential schools and what spiritual losses she sustained. We connected these losses to the capability that every individual possesses to recover spiritually once the loss has been identified. She talked about what she knew of the native healing wheel, and I researched what we did not know so we could discuss our findings in the next meeting.

---

[12] Health contracts are rarely used, but sometimes it helps to "legitimize" an agreement and cement an emotional decision. The idea is to keep this agreement in front of the client's eyes when her resolve dwindles.

Finally, I enrolled Matilde's help for Louise to know a real cancer survivor. It was an emotional meeting, wherein an instant connection was created between this wise native elder and Matilde.

It was a case of love at first sight.

Native Spirituality: My Two Worlds

I have been living in two worlds for the second half of my life, and my learning reflect this duality. Louise's case helped me to reassess my own roots as a Chilean coming from a region where the majority of the population, my family included, are coming from native roots. I became mindful of who I was and why and how I should develop this dormant spiritual perception of Gaia as the Mother Nature that nurtures and heals everything and everybody.

During my experience in working with Louise, I received a wholesome education in indigenous spirituality. Sometimes I felt very small in front of this sudden cascade of wisdom coming from this elderly Cree couple who were going through their suffering with a serene dignity, as if their sicknesses were not touching their inner soul. They taught me that acceptance of a sickness did not mean surrender to a sickness. It was a cleansing spiritual act whose outcome was left to the many spirits of nature.

An important aspect of our relationship was Louise's transformation from an elderly lady to an *elder* committed to my education in First Nations spirituality. In the many sessions we had during the four years we were working together, she taught me the difference between the way First Nations and white-man society perceive the universe.

Another finding was to realize that First Nation people carry their spirituality at all times, even if their lives have taken them to places such as prisons. While in contact with people under the Canadian Justice system, I noticed that they conserved a form of spirituality that set them apart from the rest of the population.

A First Nation person seems to be permanently immersed in his spirituality, whereas the non-indigenous population live their spiritual lives on and off or reduced them to Sunday religious practices. I am not attempting to generalize, for there must be an exception to this rule; but in what relates to aboriginal spirituality, I noticed that their spirituality has resisted assimilation from the society at large.

The same happened to "my other world," to my contact with the Mapuche nation in the southern part of Chile. During my tenure as a professor at the Temuco campus of the Universidad de Chile, part of my mandate was to conduct research and community development projects in rural areas. One of these projects was located in Repocura, a Mapuche area containing the Huentelar reserve near the town of Chol- Chol.

I was immersed in the Mapuche culture for almost two years.

In the Mapuche world, every healing activity has to comply with Mapuche spirituality, which shows an uncanny similarity with North American native beliefs (their practices mirroring Native American practices). The *Meli Witran Mapu* (the four sides of earth) is similar to the First Nation perception of the universe. There is one difference: spiritual and healing practices are mainly in the hands of a woman, the *Machi*, whose *Kultrung* (ceremonial hand drum) depicts in its design all the points of the Earth—*Piku Mapu* (north), *Willi Mapu* (south), *Puel Mapu* (east), *Lafken Mapu* (west).

The Meli Witran Mapu explains their territorial identity.

In the Mapuche social structure, the *Lonko* (Head) is the "head" of the *Lof* or community. The position can be inherited or attained by nomination from the community. The Lonko can be known as *Genpin Lonko* (in charge of the "word") or *Vlmen Lonko* (he who possesses riches) or simply Lonko (personal attribution). This is somehow similar with the Canadian First Nation's tradition in that the Chief is the head of the nation, and they respond only to a higher council of chiefs. Canadian First Nation belief system, spirituality, and healing practices are mostly in the charge of the medicine man, who seems to be like an independent practitioner with no territorial limits and no connection with the Chief.

In my Mapuche world, the Lonko heads the *Nguillatun* (a ceremony that resembles a powwow). Together with the Machi, he is in charge of keeping the traditions of the *Az Mapu* (the Mapuche land).

The Machi is a "chosen" spiritual leader in charge of health and healing. She is the intermediary between the "invisible world" and the "visible world." She communicates with both worlds through *Kvymin* or trance, which she uses to mediate with the positive and negative forces. Along with the role of spiritual leader, she is the person that knows the *Lawen* or natural medicines. She represents the *Fileu* or spirit of wisdom and healing, her power originating from a particular and defined territory; therefore, she cannot move out of her sacred territory. The clients have to come to her.

The healing ceremony is the *Machitun*, wherein the Machi heals the person or the home that has become possessed by the negative spirits.

Notable is the concept of the Fileu, the spirit that possesses the Machi even while in the maternal womb or during childhood or adolescence and communicates with her through a *Pewma* (dream). The Fileu can be received through a *Kutran* (a sickness) or a *Perimonton* (a vision).

This kind of possession through sickness and symbolic death is as well described in most texts about Shamanism. One of them written by Arnold Mindell, a Swiss psychiatrist, describes the "death walk" a shaman dreaming body experiences, wherein the person experiences the birth–death duality prior to enlightenment.

(Mindell 1993)

The Mapuche Nation, like the Cree Nation, allows only oral tradition, which is transmitted from generation to generation, allowing as well the use of trance as a form of communication with the spiritual world.

While researching the functioning of an integrated multicultural hospital in Makewe, Region de la Araucania in Chile, I received an amazing lesson from the administrator of the Makewe Hospital, who was himself a member of the Mapuche Nation.

Since it was late in the evening, I commented about the geographical position of the hospital in a hill overlooking a valley. I stated that the hospital was positioned in such a way that the patients could enjoy beautiful sunsets. Mr. Chureo, the administrator, stated that the Mapuche people never look at sunsets; they rather ignore it and consciously look at sunrises, for they gather all their energy from the birth of the day. The sun energizes everything: humans, birds, animals, plants, and trees receive the benefit of the energy of the new day. They welcome the day as part of their religious stance and thank the sun and *Nguenechen* (their Supreme Being); for they bring blessings upon the Mapuche Nation, empowering the Az Mapu and giving them the gift of a new day. The sunset represents the death of the day and the advent of darkness. Sunsets are not empowering; on the contrary, they produce a sense of despondency and sadness thus manifesting the loneliness of the Mapuche Nation.

I could not argue with this wise Lonko. Since then, I've been very mindful of my thoughts as sunrise thoughts or empowering thoughts, or as sunset thoughts or disempowering thoughts. As of today, I customarily ask the same to my clientele: are your thoughts Sunrise thoughts or Sunset thoughts?

I attempted to make some comparisons between North American First Nations and South American First Nation for the reader to note that there are more similarities than differences, even though they are worlds apart geographically. This foray into original people's medicinal and spiritual practices makes me think that perhaps traditional allopathic medicine has not learned the obvious, that many societies place a great importance in spirituality as the vehicle that moves the individual in one direction or another.

PART III

CHANGING THE PARADIGM

Conscious and Unconscious Processes and Behavioral Medicine

We have already commented that a number of physicians, like Dr. Herbert Benson from the Harvard Medical School, studied physiological changes that are produced by meditation.

Dr. Benson is the creator of the theory of the Relaxation Response. He proposed that the relaxation response is the opposite of hyperarousal and that the elicitation of the relaxation response has a positive influence on health. Hyperarousal is the state experienced when we are stressed or threatened.

Drs. Elmer and Alice Green at the Menninger Institute, Drs. David Shapiro and Gary Schwartz from Harvard, and Dr. Chandra Patel in England simultaneously researched biofeedback and self-regulation and proved that human beings could learn how to control many physiological functions through relaxation, meditation, or yoga.

Dr. Manfred Von Luhmann and Dr. Gerald Epstein utilized conscious and unconscious visualizations as a way to promote healing. Other physicians have embraced ancient Chinese healing methods, such as acupuncture. Dr. Cheek and Dr. Rossi studied the use of ideodynamic (involuntary) signalling in medical hypnosis.

All these findings have influenced the actual conceptualization of health, unanimously admitting the need of an integrative/complementary approach to health. This integrative/complementary notion states that not all knowledge is complete and must be harmonizing with models coming from other fields connected with the human environment. This larger framework known as *Behavioral Medicine*, established around 1977, is based on the premise that mind and body are intimately interconnected. Its purpose is to have a deeper understanding of health and to explore ways to promote health and disease prevention.

The Webster Medical Dictionary defines Behavioral Medicine as an "interdisciplinary field of research and practice that focuses on how people's thoughts and behavior affect their health and disease." This approach utilizes behavioral techniques such as biofeedback, relaxation training, and hypnosis.

The Journal of Psychosomatic Medicine, vol. 39, no. 6, Nov.–Dec. 1977 suggests that behavioral and psychosomatic medicine are "mostly an attitude that spouses a holistic medical practice."

Behavioral medicine releases the physician from the position of being the sole professional responsible for the patient's well-being. By way of addressing a mind-body model of treatment, this model is encouraging the patient's responsibility and is making health care more inclusive.

While the traditional model of health promotes the patient's dependence from the practitioner, the new model makes the client a member of the healing team. The client has an important role—a participative role—in his or her own healing. Cognitive, emotional, spiritual, and unconscious experiences and lifestyle factors are now considered crucial in the client's healing process.

Healing from inside out instead of relying solely in outside intervention is demonstrative of this shift.

Healing is now multidisciplinary in essence. The societal expectation of the physician as a Magi of sorts, capable of, and responsible for solving any problem, has been replaced by a more humane approach that takes away the enormous pressure deposited in this practitioner.

This shift includes the belief that including other actors from the patient's milieu, utilizing the patient's expression of his/her symptoms, and eliminating the fear of providing false expectations, can increase the effectiveness of pain management and treatment. The best example of this shift was explained to me by the family of an elderly lady who was treated by a physician from Grande Prairie in Northern Alberta.

This physician attended this elderly female patient who spoke only Spanish. The patient managed to communicate with him with some English words and hand signals, which he seemed to understand quite well. Once in a while, she would become very ill; and her physician would determine that this patient felt lonely, and her sicknesses were a way to demand attention. When she was ill, he used to communicate to the family that *Mamita* needed pampering. He admitted her to the hospital and gave instructions to the staff to provide all sorts of maneuvering in short intervals—such as blood pressure reading, small massaging, more blood pressure readings, some medication, more blood pressure and pulse taking—from early in the morning until late in the night. After two or three days of this treatment, she usually called this doctor to tell him that she felt great, that the treatment was excellent, and that she wanted to be discharged.

This plan perfectly addressed the needs of this patient—who, by the way, had an amazing capacity to somatise her emotional needs—transforming them into heart conditions symptoms, high blood pressure readings, rheumatoid arthritis, and digestive problems.

Behavioral medicine seems to be evolving toward the actual integrative model that places the individual suffering from ill health as an active member of the team. This model of medicine does not separate the individual from his context, rather it incorporates this milieu as an important element in the healing process.

Basic Approaches to Therapeutic Healing

The Therapist-Client Relationship

In any treatment, the relationship between therapist and client follows two basic approaches that define the outcome of the treatment: the nonparticipant approach and the active participant approach (in the healing process). Both approaches are beautifully illustrated in two books. The first one relates the battle of a promising athlete who decided to dedicate his remaining time to help children, dying a hero a year and a half after his diagnosis of melanoma.

The second book describes the case of a writer who decided, after a six-month-to-live prognosis due to a metastasized melanoma, to search for a treatment that suited her needs and beliefs. She was in remission after eighteen months of treatment, almost the identical time that took for the athlete of the first book to die. The books are *A Shining Season* by William Buchanan, published by Bantam Books, and *My Triumph over Cancer* by Beata Bishop, published by Keats Publishing.

The nonparticipant approach describes the relationship between patient and practitioner as one of dependency and passive participation, wherein the patient deposits total responsibility of the treatment in the hands of the practitioner. The patient's role is to receive medical attention; and their only participation is as a consumer of services, a recipient of goods. The patient has only to follow the directions given for their treatment, and their input is either minimal or non-existent.

The active participant approach is the one that allows the client to take a proactive role in his own treatment by accepting full responsibility for his sickness and recovery. I am using the term client as a synonym of active participation, as opposed to patient or nonparticipant individual. This is the approach that I have endorsed in my work with the sometimes unjustly labeled terminally ill clients.

There are many client-centred approaches, and all of them have something in common. The common approach is the amount of responsibility placed in the client's capabilities to generate their own experience, reframe their old experiences, and be in the therapy. The role of the therapist is to empower this client with a feeling of control and trust, to avoid imposing unwarranted demands, and to provide guidance and information on how to reframe and transform pathological experiences.

Rossi states that "patients have problems because of learned limitations. They have developed conscious mindsets that inhibit their conscious problem-solving efforts." (Erickson 1992, p. 89)

Even if the therapist is purposely guiding the client's attention in a given direction, the therapist must provide an alternative path toward the objective. Clients should feel that they have the freedom of choice, the freedom to respond in a manner that is comfortable and organic; and they should be reassured that their responses are good. The feeling of freedom is one of the most pleasant and comforting feelings, and the therapist should convey this feeling continuously. (Havens 1985, p. 168)

Self-management interventions have been used successfully in the treatment of anxiety, depression, and pain. Even though I wholeheartedly endorse self- management care, it has been my experience that it is always more effective for the clients to have another person coaching them in their self-managed treatment. Self-hypnosis is recommended in many books, and it is a true healing tool; however, for a client in pain and in fear, it is almost impossible to acquire the detachment from symptoms that is required for self-hypnosis to be successful. It can be used at a level in which recovery is practically achieved and self-hypnosis is used as reinforcement; but in the initial stage of problem solving, coaching is a must.

Mind-body Models of Clinical Intervention

One of the models that I have been using in combination with the trance state is the Mind-body Model of Dr. Carl Simonton, an oncologist from Bridgeport, Texas. He developed a model that in many aspects mirrors the one developed by the Harvard Mind-body Institute. Both models point toward interventions with not only cancer or HIV/AIDS patients, but also additionally encompassing every psychosomatic illness present nowadays in our stressed-out society. The Simonton Model provides a theoretical and practical framework for the therapist to follow, and it can be described as a comprehensive cognitive–behavioral self-help therapy designed to help the cancer sufferer and the people involved in their support system. It encompasses the emotional, cognitive, behavioral, social, and spiritual aspect of human existence. It can be delivered as an individual therapy, as well as a group modality.

I found this approach easier to implement and easier to explain to clients. Utilizing the books written by Dr. Simonton as reference material allows my clients to understand and to follow Dr. Simonton's healing protocol successfully.

My therapeutic approach follows these models. I routinely favor the incorporation of a dietician to have the client well covered in every angle. I am sold on the value of exercising whenever possible because it complements the election of a proper diet.

I make a point of using psycholinguistics[13] and medical hypnosis in cancer treatments because in my opinion, they are the best and fastest ways to produce significant changes in my client's preparedness to heal. These methods allow me to access the unconscious maps contained in the state-dependent information and learning. By engaging their unconscious mind, I access their brain's GPS, which will guide them in the road toward recovery.

Our unconscious mind is a tireless worker that controls all the functions of the bodymind on a 24/7 basis. Whether asleep

---

[13] Psycholinguistics explains the relationship between thinking and the processing of language by the brain. It explains the processes that make possible to generate meaningful sentences and to understand ideas. (Author's note)

or awake, it controls the heart and lung functions, digestive and glandular processes, etc. Additionally, this unconscious mind modulates cellular activity with total independence from our conscious mind.

In 1984, Pert and Ruff were already researching macrophage mutation in the lungs as a response of toxicity in the environment, explaining that these mutations were produced by a hyper-response of the immune system in the form of sending in macrophages in great quantities. These macrophages, working overtime, mutated into cancer cells that metastasized all over the body. Concurrently, they discovered that the same peptides found in the brain were found in the immune system as well therefore suggesting intercommunication among the mind, the immune system, and the endocrine system. This psycho-immuno-endrocrine network was the initial step in the creation of the field of psychoneuroimmunology (PNI). (Pert 1984, pp. 169–171)

The importance of these developments is that it confirms beyond doubt that the mind and the central nervous system regulate (modulate) cellular activity.

Ernest Lawrence Rossi, PhD, describes three stages in this modularity:

Stage One. Mind-generated thoughts and imagery (neural impulses) are created in the frontal cortex.

Stage Two. These mind-generated impulses are filtered through the state-dependent memory and learning and emotional areas of the limbic–hypothalamic system and transduced into the neurotransmitters that regulate the organs of the autonomic nervous system, which branches into the sympathetic (activating) and parasympathetic (relaxing) systems. Both systems in turn secrete the neurotransmitters norepinephrine and acetylcholine to initiate the next stage.

Stage Three. Information is transduced[14] (changed over) by the neurotransmitters to the organs by binding with the receptor in

---

[14]   Transduction is the process whereby a transducer (a devise that convert energy into something different) accepts energy in one form and gives back related energy in a different form.

their cell walls, changing in the process its molecular structure, or by activating an enzyme in the cell membrane to create a process of communication involving adenylcyclase and the resulting adenosine triphosphate (ATP) and cyclic adenosine monophosphate (CAMP). This explanation serves the purpose to illustrate the notion that "mind modulates the biochemical functions within the cells of all the major organs systems and tissues of the body via the autonomic nervous system." (Rossi's emphasis in Rossi 1984, pp. 107–108)

For years I have been involved in researching the effectiveness of hypnotic communication in mind-body modulation and the altered states of consciousness as the ground where healing battles are won and lost. My findings suggest that there is no reason to shy away from attempting to manipulate neurotransmitters modularity into influencing tissue regeneration in cancer cases. If emotions have specific biochemical correlates[15] influencing sickness and health, we could utilize these emotions to influence this modularity toward health and tissue regeneration. When explaining to colleagues the possibility to utilize trance and psycholinguistic techniques to modulate the mind, I realize that sometimes their position as employees of a system (e.g., hospital, clinic, government health department, etc.) did not allow them to take advantage of the opportunities to try something different. Many institutions forbid their professionals to use therapeutic approaches other than cognitive–behavioral models, which are equated to "evidence-based" models. Even if there is ample scientific evidence of biochemical correlates influencing mind modularity, hypnotherapy is still unrecognized as one of the most effective tools for mindbody modularity.

While listening to the instructors in the Mind-body Medicine and the Relaxation Response at Harvard Medical School, talking about the effectiveness of yoga and meditation in the treatment of psychosomatic illnesses, I could not avoid the thought that if we push beyond the relaxation response and provide a direction for the

---

15   Correlates are two or more related or complementary elements found in a biochemical reaction. (Author's note)

relaxation state, we could connect with state-dependent memory and learning to influence psychoneural modulation of oncogenic growth factors[16] into cancer remission.

The Simonton Model of Cancer Development and Recovery

Cancer Development Model

I like Dr. Simonton's model of cancer development because is easy to understand, and it is consonant with the findings of all the practitioners that are supporting the Non-dual medicine concept. This integral model of cancer development outlines a step-by-step generation and progression of the sickness based on the existing evidence that stress predisposes people to sickness. The Simonton's cognitive reframing regards cancer cells as weak and confused and the immune system's cells as powerful and destructive. This type of visualization lowers the influence of fear networks and empowers the client toward health by visualizing the immune system's cells as an all-destructive force with the power to annihilate the confused and not-so-intelligent cancer cells. (Simonton 1992)

My wife, Matilde, visualized her immune system NK[17] cells as knights in shiny armour riding white horses and destroying those crab-like creatures representing her cancer cells. I do not know how to measure the effectiveness of such visualization, other than realizing that Matty has used the same visualization to already destroy three cancers in twenty-nine (29) years. She is still *living with* and not *fighting* her cancers. She does not need more evidence or proof than that, and I am not prepared to contradict this lady master destroyer.

According to Dr. Simonton, despair, hopelessness, and depression impair our coping mechanisms; and consciously and

---

16   Genetic alteration of cells is produced by elements or signals called growth factors.

17   Natural Killer cell is a cytotoxic lymphocyte, a major player of the innate immune system to respond to infections and fighting tumors. (Author's notes)

unconsciously, we perceive death as a potential solution to our problems.

This mindset is acknowledged by the limbic system, which records these feelings of despair and hopelessness. The information is sent to the hypothalamus, which translates it in messages to destabilize and weaken the immune system, thus deregulating the pituitary gland. As a consequence, the endocrine system is compromised; and an imbalance in adrenal hormones makes the body susceptible to carcinogenic substances.

Researchers have studied how the immune system responds in people who "feel lonely" (Vanderhaeghe 1999, p. 87). These people perceive

themselves as trapped in situations that may be perceived differently by others. They feel their situation as real; and as such, they unconsciously allow their immune system to decline, making them vulnerable to disease. The same authors are of the opinion that loneliness is a major factor in immune suppression and requires an examination of our emotional being to "reboot" our immune system.

This might explain counselling and membership in support groups increasing the client's capability to combat sicknesses.

Other than loneliness, there are many toxic emotions having the capability of destabilizing our immune system. Feeling angry and enraged, sad, depressed, afraid or terrified, helpless, confused, frustrated, inadequate, embarrassed or ashamed will make us susceptible to illnesses.

Psychologists already realized that people born with disabilities were better adjusted than people that acquired disabilities later in life. The effect of these disabilities not only affects the individual, but also their milieu. Relatives, friends, and associates feel the same pain, the same frustration, and the same anxiety as the affected individual.

Viruses are important culprits in the generation of certain cancers. Helicobacter Pylori may be the cause of stomach cancer; Human T-Cell Lymphoma virus has been syndicated as the cause of T-Cell Lymphoma; Papilloma virus was connected to cervical cancer, etc.

At the base of these sicknesses, there is always the weakening of the immune system that allows these viruses to circumvent our body's defenses.

In prior chapters, I mentioned the work of Manfred Von Luhmann and John Selby, who researched the healing process and its relationship with the state of mind of individuals who were ill or injured. They noticed a tendency to spend time thinking about the past or reflecting about the future and spending very little time in the present, which is the slice of time in which the sickness or injury manifests itself. In the opinion of both scientists, the focus of attention should be the immediate present—the here and now—when the body needs total concentration to heal.

Von Luhmann and Selby suggest the following basic rules to solve this problem:

-The patient must keep their attention focused in the present to encourage immune system activation. Focusing in the future or in the past does very little to activate their bodies' self defenses.

-Since breathing is in the present, by focusing on their breathing, the client can tune into the here and now, which is the time when healing takes place.

-Another way to focus in the present is to concentrate on the beating of the heart and on body motion thus bringing to consciousness unconscious processes, such as walking or using muscles to achieve and maintain balance.

Jon Kabat-Zinn is actively researching mindfulness-based stress reduction and its utilization in a wide spectrum of maladies grouped under the umbrella of pain and suffering, which deepens Von Luhmann and Selby's model.

Mind-body Model of Recovery

Dr. O. Carl Simonton's mind-body model of recovery reverses the previously outlined model of sickness using the same pathway. Feelings are utilized to change physiological conditions by strengthening the client's beliefs that they have a degree of control over the outcome of the sickness.

If the weakening of the immune system produces the sickness, the contrary is equally true. We potentiate our body's defenses through changing our beliefs and eliminating stress-generating situations. Beliefs in recovery generate feelings of hope, which in turn are recorded in the limbic system in the same way that the stressors were recorded. These feelings of hope are sent to the hypothalamus, which in turn sends messages to the pituitary gland. These new messages mobilize, once again, the body's defenses.

The hormonal balance is once again restored. (Simonton 1992)

Years ago I Met Dr. Mariusz Wirga and since then, I have maintained some form of communication with him.

Dr. Wirga is the Medical Director of Psychosocial Oncology at the Todd Cancer Institute in Long Beach Memorial Medical Centre, Long Beach, California. He is furthering the work of Dr. Simonton who died on June 18, 2009.

We met while attending the 2010 IPOS convention in Quebec. He kindly sent me an excerpt of his correspondence about Dr. Simonton's work that I trust will be a great help to further Dr. Simonton's cancer program.

Dr. Wirga stated the following:

Since Dr. Simonton first published the results of his work, there were four randomized clinical trials (David Spiegel, Fawzy Fawzy, Thomas Kuchler, and Barbara Andersen) showing improved survival for cancer patients receiving appropriate psychotherapy in conjunction with conventional cancer treatment.

Frequently his contribution to medicine is identified with a corrupted form of simplistic understanding of visualization or mental imagery. As a matter of fact, I don't remember him using the word "visualization" since we first met in 1990. For Dr. Simonton, imagery was a natural process occurring in our minds all the time. His most frequent example of imagery was asking the audience "What did you have for breakfast?" He emphasized that we are all experts at using our imagery in our own way. Try to sit for a few seconds and not to imagine anything. Impossible (unless you are a master of particular meditative practices with dozens of years of daily multihour experience). Carl considered the content and quality of these cognitions to be the key for health. He developed a very sophisticated approach to shift these thoughts in a healthy direction and refined imagery exercises that were individualized to the particular style, symbolism, and needs of a person. His patients are becoming experts at using their continuous natural imagery in healthy ways to promote getting well.

Furthermore, the Simonton Program—as it is taught in USA, Japan, Poland, Germany, Italy, and Holland— is a very comprehensive approach and goes far beyond the use of imagery. Dr. Simonton was the first one to introduce cognitive–behavior therapy (CBT) to psychosocial oncology (with the help of Dr. Maxie C. Maultsby), and now CBT is a standard part of the treatment in psycho-oncology. The Simonton Program systematically addresses multiple issues that cancer patients and their families deal with, like fatigue and low energy, relationships and communication problems, recognizing patterns of stress and secondary gains, resolving spiritual and personal philosophical challenges, as well as integrating life with death and maintaining healthy hope in all stages of treatment.

> *The Program employs multiple therapeutic modalities including individual, group, and family therapies, behavioral (relaxation, balancing a healthy lifestyle with exercise, nutrition, and play), cognitive (CBT and education), mindfulness, resolving guilt and resentment, improving compliance with cancer treatments by developing healthier beliefs about them and seeing them as friends and allies. This is the only psychosocial oncology program in continuous operation since 1971. Dr. Simonton kept at advancing and refining his approach to the last day of his life, so let's not limit it just to imagery and peg it to old clichés.*[18]

In summary, this model of cancer creation and recovery acknowledges the existence of unconscious resources that can produce health as well as sicknesses; therefore, an important part of the intervention must be geared toward changing unconscious patterns of behavior—which requires, as might be expected from the practitioner, to work with the encrypted messages contained in the unconscious mind. Technology allows the physician to locate the problem areas. My role is to create in this client an appropriate mindset to activate the body's own defenses by adding feelings and beliefs for wellness to the medical equation.

By adding the human dimension and by treating the body and the mind as an indivisible unit, we make a huge difference in the outcome of any treatment.

From the colon cancer in room number 24 (the patient has become his cancer, losing in the process his own identity), you revert back into Mr. Shane Smith, a patient suffering from cancer.

---

[18] Correspondence sent to me by Dr. Wirga to clarify some of Dr. Simonton's concepts after his death. (Published with author's permission.)

IMPLEMENTING THE INFORMATION

Wilber's Integral Theory

For years I have been attempting to create a frame or a system to organize the distinct yet connected parts of my clinical approach in my work with clients suffering from cancer. For the sake of visualizing the healing process, the idea of creating a structure and a picture of the therapeutic interaction of the client and the practitioner have been present in my mind to create something simple, easy to visualize that could encompass everything . . . something we could put up on a wall to represent the individual, the practitioner, the family, and the social resources. A system encompassing methods and what is available in the society—or in the universe, for that matter—to help the client to achieve recovery.

While researching this possibility, I discovered Wilber's Integral Quadrant Theory. His "Theory of Everything" is, in my opinion, a perfect map, a perfect step-by-step construct that is instrumental in organizing the information. Wilber's quadrants helped me to visualize the road to sickness, as well as the road to recovery.

Wilber is not an easy reading, and his degree of complexity might discourage some from taking the time to read (and understand) this young philosopher's writings. I am attempting to simplify some of his ideas and, in the process, ask for forgiveness; for this part might be a little bit academic.

Wilber's designs include the subjective and the objective world of the client and the practitioner, as well as the subjective and objective resources that are available for healing and recovery for both of them, the individual and collective world of the client as well as the procedures and institutions involved in the healing and recovery process. I have to remind myself that when an individual is sick, the whole society also suffers with this sickness.

Wilber's Quadrants

My goal is to "operationalize" a procedure through the use of systems contained in Wilber's Integral Theory, purposely avoiding explaining his philosophy. Instead, I would like to invite the reader to peruse the many excellent books written by Ken Wilber. My present goal is to use his map to create a working model for cancer interpretation and recovery. In a nutshell, Wilber created four quadrants to encompass anything that is connected with the client. It is, therefore, an integral and integrative view of a client, his very personal circumstances, his connection with the world, and his position in the world. The same quadrants also show the individual and collective world of the therapist in intimate connection with the client's quadrants. They represent the therapist universe— his values and personal situation in connection with the client, his treatment modalities and techniques, his connection with a larger reality that supports his professional endeavour (such as the institution to which he belongs and in which way both client and therapist connects with society).

Wilber artfully explains the upper-left-hand dimension of the quadrant—which is dedicated to the interior human dimension, the soul, the spirit, and the beliefs of client and practitioner alike. It is the subjective aspect of consciousness and individual awareness. The language of this quadrant is "I". It is the way "I" see my reality. It is my perception of things.

I see my own intention, the reason behind my effort, the purpose that guides my intention to do healing work while defining myself as a member of a larger community. In the same way, I am asking my client to define himself/herself to apply her most honest effort to define who she is, why she feels this way, and what the guiding principles behind her purpose or lack of energy to concentrate on healing and recovery are.

The upper left is a complete portrait of my client—what he thinks, what he believes, what he feels. It is also my portrait—my life and professional purpose, beliefs, limitations, skills, feelings, strengths, weaknesses, etc. All of it are in connection with the problem situation that the client is bringing to me in my role as a specialist or as a practitioner.

The lower-left-hand quadrant, also part of the subjective realm, is the "WE" realm. It is the collective that embraces the individual and the cultural environment containing Mores, Folkways, values, moral, and ethics regulating the connection of the individual with the society.

I belong to a church, to a group of individuals, to a family, to a club, to a belief. I am a Shaman belonging to a group that thinks in the same way. I follow the group or societal principles that support my philosophical being. In my role as a practitioner, I belong to my client's world and "we" are embracing the same intention toward health and healing, working as a team toward explaining and solving problems.

The upper-right-hand quadrant represents the realm of the "IT", the objective, the exterior physical tools of an individual, the individual's interior consciousness. It is the body, the brain, the bodymind expressed in its organic parts. It also represents the mechanisms, the actions we develop to solve the problems of the "SELF," the individual's scientific part, the concepts forming part of the brain, and the method used for problem-solving (including brain mechanisms and communication substances that create the red of communication of the bodymind, as well as the inclusion of individual competencies that the self possesses for problem-solving and adaptation).

I believe that at any point, we are bombarded by eleven million pieces of information, out of which we can process only forty pieces of information; therefore, I concentrate my efforts on the most informed module, which is the unconscious module. I customarily use methods such as the Simonton Method, Ericksonian Hypnotherapy, and trance toward modulation of immune response. My client brings to the equation what he/she knows about his/her sickness and what he/she thinks should be done to restore trust, hope, and health, bringing as well the many personal tools for healing contained in her very personal tool crib.

The lower-right-hand quadrant represents the "ITS", the collective medium in which the other three quadrants float—organizations, brick and mortar institutions, clinics, schools, and social systems that regulate the actions of the three quadrants.

I practice at an institution, clinic, office. I belong to the societal health system. I am connected with hospitals, insurance systems, and colleges that regulate my relationship with my client. I am a member of a society, of a country, and of an international organization.

While attempting to utilize Wilber's philosophy and methods, I am well aware that this is quite a simplified approach that in no way explains Wilber; rather, I am utilizing some of his tenets—which, in my opinion, can provide a very encompassing map to treat not only cancer, but also every mind-body ailment.

The common denominator connecting healers and healing efforts is the quest to bring about change, to grow and develop as human beings while creating at the same time a working model for integral health and healing.

Wilber talks about the three eyes of knowing that every human being has: the eye of flesh, the eye of the mind, and the eye of contemplation. The first one is connected with empiricism. It is the one that is connected to science and examines something that is evident (2+2=4).

The second one, the eye of the mind, is connected with logical thought, with reason, and with what our brain is telling us about what we are observing.

The third one, the eye of contemplation, is connected with emotions and spirit. It is connected with the way we react in front of somebody's suffering. It is the way we filter experiences through our values and beliefs. These three eyes of knowing give us a complete, integral view of what is observed (Wilber 1998).

Anything observed through only one or two filters will give us an incomplete, faulty, and monological view of what is observed.

These three modes of inquiry, in my opinion, form the base of non-dual medicine.

In one of his comments, Wilber amazingly seems to describe the role of the therapist:

> Thus you might see me coming down the street, a frown on my face. You can see that. But what does that exterior frown actually mean? How you will find out? You will ask me. You will talk to me. You can see my surfaces, but in order to understand my interior, my depths, you will have to enter into the interpretive circle. You, as a subject, will not merely stare at me as an object (of the monological gaze); rather, you, as a subject, will attempt to understand me as a subject, as a person, as a self, as a bearer of intentionality and meaning. You will talk to me and interpret what I say, and I will do the same with you. We are not subjects staring at objects; we are subjects trying to understand subjects. We are in the intersubjective circle, the dialogical dance. Monological is to describe; dialogical is to understand . . . to put it bluntly, exterior surfaces can be seen, but interior depth must be interpreted. (Wilber 1998, p. 118)

Another important element to take into consideration in the implementation of treatment is the difference between a *method* and a *process*.

A method is an algorithm to be used to achieve a goal, a construct that contains sets of beliefs and procedures to be used to achieve a defined goal or goals, a structure containing principles within which change is defined and "operationalized."

A process is the way in which we "operationalize" the transformation we want to achieve, which is defined in the method.

In my work with my clients, I support the use of the four quadrants and the "Transcend and Include Development Method" created by Ken Wilber because they allow me to include other methods and procedures (such as the Simonton Method, the Freire's Method, and Dr. Benson's Relaxation Response) that, in my opinion, are valid in the resolution of the many problems and issues that the clientele bring to our office. The Wilber Method *transcends* the present situation of the client but *includes* what is transcended in the therapeutic process as valuable information. Clients *transcend* the level where they are via the experience gained through the pain and suffering that brought this client to seek the help of a therapist. We do not dismiss the information; we process and transform this energy into knowledge and information that will be the basis for transformation.

The value of Wilber's Quadrants resides in its capacity to encompass everything thus creating an integrative picture of the client and of the therapist, both interacting in a therapeutic relationship. Wilber asserts that "awareness in and of itself is curative" and that "every therapeutic school attempts to allow consciousness to encounter facets of experience that were previously alienated, malformed, distorted or ignored" (Wilber 2000, p. 99). Awareness can be attained only as a consequence of an inquiry into the state-dependent contents of the unconscious mind. Making the unconscious conscious is the preceding step to attaining awareness. The healing value of these experiences resides in the possibility to observe them from the outside, to see them as objects, and thus explore and reframe these contents to attain health.

Wilber's Basic Four Quadrants

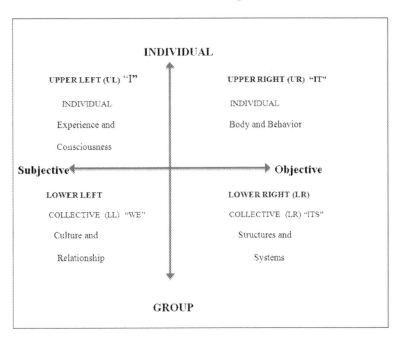

When I "operationalize" the quadrants by adding the procedures, it looks like this:

Individual

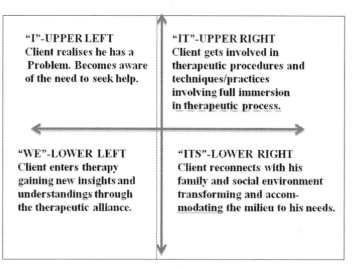

"I"-UPPER LEFT Client realises he has a Problem. Becomes aware of the need to seek help.	"IT"-UPPER RIGHT Client gets involved in therapeutic procedures and techniques/practices involving full immersion in therapeutic process.
"WE"-LOWER LEFT Client enters therapy gaining new insights and understandings through the therapeutic alliance.	"ITS"-LOWER RIGHT Client reconnects with his family and social environment transforming and accommodating the milieu to his needs.

Group (collective)

The advantage of Wilber's method is that it provides a map for treatment that is encompassing of every therapeutic modality. Each quadrant represents a specific dimension of the individual, as well as the relationships this individual creates within the society. It also represents the different tools this individual uses to communicate with his milieu. Additionally, it allows the practitioner to examine the client's *present state of being*. This present-to-future paradigm has the purpose to make sure that the "current me" will allow the "new me" to grow.

The present state of being (PSOB) represents what has to transcend and include to become the "new state of being" (NSOB), the new level created by the information obtained from the old experience.

The present state of being is the client's manifestation in the world: the Self, Subject, or "I." It is the subject with whom the therapist works, the subject that is to transcend through therapy into the new state of being. Once the NSOB is established as a new level of being, it becomes the new starting point for a new level.

This is a process that involves a constant and never-ending motion of PSOB transforming into a NSOB with all of this taking place within the frame of the four quadrants.

Once the therapeutic alliance is established within the realm of the Upper Left and Lower left, my client and I move into the Upper Right quadrant and utilize a combination of the Simonton Model, the Selye's Model, and the Harvard Mind-body Model. As an addition to these models, I incorporate the use of trance states to amplify the effect of changework and to enhance in the client the belief that recovery is possible (UL). I am also incorporating tenets of the Consciousness Raising Methods of Paulo Freire (LR), which were briefly explained while discussing Louise's case.

Laura Divine™, a very skilled Integral coach, explains the four-quadrants lens with great clarity. I am including them in an effort to clarify even further the dynamics of the quadrants.

SUBJECTIVE   **INDIVIDUAL**   **OBJECTIVE**

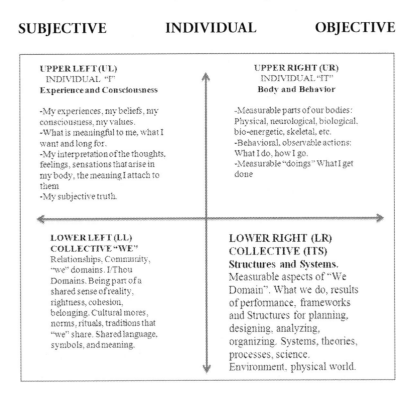

UPPER LEFT (UL)	UPPER RIGHT (UR)
INDIVIDUAL "I"	INDIVIDUAL "IT"
Experience and Consciousness	**Body and Behavior**
-My experiences, my beliefs, my consciousness, my values.	-Measurable parts of our bodies: Physical, neurological, biological, bio-energetic, skeletal, etc.
-What is meaningful to me, what I want and long for.	-Behavioral, observable actions: What I do, how I go.
-My interpretation of the thoughts, feelings, sensations that arise in my body, the meaning I attach to them	-Measurable "doings" What I get done
-My subjective truth.	
LOWER LEFT (LL)	**LOWER RIGHT (LR)**
COLLECTIVE "WE"	**COLLECTIVE (ITS)**
Relationships, Community, "we" domains. I/Thou Domains. Being part of a shared sense of reality, rightness, cohesion, belonging. Cultural mores, norms, rituals, traditions that "we" share. Shared language, symbols, and meaning.	**Structures and Systems.** Measurable aspects of "We Domain". What we do, results of performance, frameworks and Structures for planning, designing, analyzing, organizing. Systems, theories, processes, science. Environment, physical world.

L. Divine™ 2009.Journal of Integral Theory and Practice-Vol.4, N0. 1.

Published with author's authorization.

As I mentioned before, I am incorporating into the quadrants (LR) Paulo Freire's Consciousness Raising Method, which he developed initially for literacy programs.

I like to use this method because it allows for the embodiment of an individual's/actor's own personal history, as well as the acquisition of awareness of his rights and responsibilities and the promotion of personal growth.

We are already aware that healing takes place in the very moment when the client discovers and internalizes the notion that they are actors in their own recovery.

Empowerment and embodiment are the expected logical outputs of consciousness raising methods. Embodiment is conceptualized as a knowledge that becomes natural to the "body." It is something that is accepted and incorporated naturally into our "self."

Traditionally the client is or becomes a "patient," somebody that has a problem and has no control over it. In a "patient" concept of the world, the control lies on the practitioner who sees the "patient" as a simple receptor of the benefit of his knowledge and skills. This patient has no opinion and is subjected to the maneuvering of a whole system that does not take into consideration his feelings, emotions, and experiences. The patient's personal experience is disregarded as unimportant, and all the decisions are in the hands of physicians and nurses who "know better" about what the patient needs than the patient himself. The patient's whole persona has no medical value other than being the body that is the object of the practitioner's maneuvering.

Treatment is delivered as if the patient is simply a *sick body*.

Implicit in this concept is the assumption that the patient has no knowledge of his own problem and is "in the world" as an object of a system which dehumanizes and devalues him.

A while ago, at a hospital in Edmonton, Alberta, I witnessed a physician talking to a female patient recently diagnosed with cancer of the liver. When the patient stated that she needed to see her biopsy information to fight this cancer, he said "Everything inside of you is terrible . . . terrible! And no one surgeon in Edmonton is going to touch you . . . You have about three months to live." Obviously this physician thought that his opinion and his time were too important to be wasted in listening to this patient wanting to fight back and survive. To my surprise, he added . . . "I cannot show you the biopsy information because it went missing between the first and fifth floor, but I was told that everything is terrible . . . terrible." To my question of whether he read the pathologist report or not, he stated that he did not, (but) . . . "I was informed that the report cannot show whether there is or not cancer in the back portion of the liver, but I am pretty sure that it is full of cancer." To my question whether surgery could be possible even if they did not know the extension of the metastasis or not, he stated that it was not possible but that he was not sure.

I could notice how unconcerned and uninformed this physician was. The client was at the mercy of this practitioner, and predictably, she subsequently refused any form of treatment.

She died a month and a half after this interview.

I feel relieved by realizing that in my experience working with dedicated physicians, this is an exception, not the rule.

Opposing this vision is the notion of a fully informed client, a person that is cognizant (not a cognizable object,) a person that feels liberated and is a part of the act of cognition. The client is no longer at the end of the cognitive act but is an able and active participant in his life, an actor in his own process. Both practitioner and client become mutually responsible for the act of healing and recovery. Through the dialogue, practitioner and client cease to exist as individuals, emerging instead as equal partners engaged in the process of attaining health and freedom from a system that de-personalizes them.

It is indeed a transformational act of health.

This is what is at the base of the practitioner's transformational praxis, which can be also incorporated into a group therapy model.

Freire's notion of culture circles sees each participant as a dynamic unit interacting with the coordinator (in this case, the therapist) through a dialogical communication—analysing, de-codifying, and re-codifying the experience—and acting upon these new codifications (reframing). The group teaches the individual the ways and means to change a pathological perception of reality for one predominantly critical and informed. The Freire's Method is a typical example of the integral use of the four quadrants.

Critical understanding leads to critical action; pathological understanding leads to pathological responses. Critical understanding can be achieved through an active, dialogical, horizontal relationship with the client, using a personal, idiosyncratic matrix and involving the client's thematic and vocabular universe.

The Freire's Method sees the role of the participant as not merely being in the world, but actively engaging in relations with the world, which is translated into an active and egalitarian participation in the therapeutic process.

Other experiences involving individuals and milieu are described by Bill Moyers, a journalist who interviewed several professionals supporting Mind-body Medicine. One of them, David Smith, MD, (a Commissioner of the Texas Department of Health) describes his clinical work as a "Community-Oriented Primary Care Clinic." He describes his experiences with ethnic communities that have a precarious access to the American Health System, as well as describing the relationship with health and mindbody medicine. He states that every aspect of an illness has a component that relates to mind and that, in any healing process, the mind is very intricately involved with whether the client gets better or worse. To Dr. Smith, every cultural model is relevant in the healing process and the use of community workers allow the individuals to see sickness and healing as a responsibility of a whole milieu. In this system, in order for the individual to have a feeling of control over his own sickness, information is paramount. Every individual has the right to know what is happening to his body, as well as the right to make decisions about it.

Another professional utilizing a similar approach as Freire and Smith is Jon Kabat-Zinn. His patients at his stress reduction clinic seat themselves in a circle (on the floor or in folding chairs) and meditate while using mind-concentrating techniques, such as slowly eating raisins. This is part of a body-scanning technique, which Kabat-Zinn calls Mindfulness. The same method (this time a circle of women suffering from breast cancer) has at its center a psychiatrist named David Spiegel. The place is Stanford University, and Spiegel is conducting a research that is based on his statement that the right mental attitude can help a patient to conquer cancer. He also stated "The sense of social alienation that many cancer patients suffer . . . is a terrible thing and a danger to their mental and physical health" (Moyers 1993, p. 79).

Dean Ornish, another mind-body physician, has managed to reverse heart disease in patients by only using the power of their minds, a low-fat diet, and moderate exercise.

In the examples outlined above, the common denominator is the level of integrity that is associated with a process that sees the client/patient as a full participant/actor in the healing process.

As you can see, there are many things that can be placed on the proper quadrant: information, reflections, notes, procedures, theories, etc. Given any particular information that might be useful to the practitioner, the client can be contained in the specific quadrant.

This is what Wilber calls his "Theory of Everything."

PART IV

STAGES OF TREATMENT

Upper Left, and Lower Left Quadrants

UPPER LEFT (UL) **INDIVIDUAL "I"** Experience and Consciousness	
LOWER LEFT (LL) **COLLECTIVE "WE"** Culture and Relationships	

The Upper Left "I" and Lower Left "WE" quadrants or lenses are the subjective parts of the equation and contain the practitioner's individual experiences—as well as the client's experiences, beliefs, values, and interpretation of their respective worlds, coupled with thoughts, feelings, and life meanings. The lower left quadrant includes family and close relationships, culture, language, and societal norms (professional ethics regulating the practitioner–client relationship, etc.).

The First Five Minutes

One of the most common mistakes we make as practitioners is to dismiss the client's feelings of fear and pain as unimportant, or worse, imaginary.

Whatever the client is experiencing is true to him and therefore legitimate.

By acknowledging and legitimizing these feelings, we convey to the client an empowering message of trust and support, inviting him to utilize all his emotional resources to strengthen the healing alliance, which is paramount to the continuance and success of the treatment.

The client will notice that this practitioner possesses the sensibility required to understand the problem and the flexibility to position and to observe the problem from the client's perspective. Consequently, the client will feel and judge that this practitioner can be trusted.

Traditional healing practices suggest that practitioners should detach their feelings from those of the client. Sometimes the practitioner talks with the client from behind a desk, which immediately creates a barrier. I posit that the practitioner should even go to the point of sharing personal experiences that are connected with the client's situation. This has to be done with tact and within the rules of privilege of information. The objective is to create, in the first five minutes, commonality and a strong rapport, which is a sine-qua-non condition to the establishment of a healing alliance. This alliance will allow the practitioner to obtain important, relevant, and detailed information that will provide the parameters to formulate a treatment plan. The client's narrative will provide information that can be used to reframe negative experiences and to create metaphors for unconscious changework.

Once the client accepts the practitioner as a person willing and capable of understanding the problem, changework is promoted even deeper.

The next step in this first meeting is to obtain the permission from the patient to create a set of therapeutic tools for therapeutic use.

We have to remember that the client must be empowered with the responsibility to plan, in partnership with the practitioner, his or her own treatment. Once this objective is achieved, a contract for a number of sessions—as well as clarification of practitioner and client's roles—should be discussed.

The client must have a clear understanding that treatment and healing cannot take place in the absence of full cooperation and mutual trust.

The therapist should be aware that the client might be unconsciously using him/her as a role model.

Once the client and the practitioner settle for the healing contract, the first question to address is the essential question of meaning:

How important is it for you to heal (live)?

This question is formulated to obtain a maximum amount of information regarding client's motivation, as well as identifying the generative themes to be used to place the focus on the important themes that motivate the client to heal.

I customarily use *heal* instead of *live* or *survive*. These two words, I found, have a negative connotation because they generate a sense of fear to the whole process. It is better to use words connected with hope and success and devoid of threatening overtones. When I use healing, I also add to the client's unconscious mind the notion of not healing, which has a lesser negative meaning than the concept of surviving, which automatically brings into the client's mind its own opposite: dying.

It is important to emphasise that while we are gathering information from a client, we are also making sure that the information gathered is rich in content, vocabular modalities, and ideas as expressed by the client. It is important to collect as much information as possible, especially key sentences and values expressed in certain words that are idiosyncratic to the client. We have to harvest the client's unique vocabular and thematic universe, main ideas, values, images, and metaphors with the purpose of creating a linguistic bank of information to produce meaningful messages via the utilization of vocabulary, contents, and values expressed by the client. This is the way to produce changes in their unconscious maps through the use of utterances that have special value to them, expressed with the same vocabulary that they use to describe their condition, feelings, and experiences.

A second set of generative themes can be identified through the following question:

What are you planning to do once you recover your health?

The answer to this question will provide us with the action or actions that have to be programmed in order to set in motion the principles contained in the first set of themes, which relate to the most important reasons the client has to heal (survive). Through this question, we are also projecting the client toward a hopeful future. The answers generated by this question will also provide us with detailed information about hopes and expectations. Contents will be used to create the messages (and an alternative mind roadmap) that set the plan into motion. It will serve the purpose to review, revise, and re-discuss treatment objectives with the client whenever his/her resolve dwindles.

This is the stage of hope.

As stated before, instillation of hope is what makes the difference between fight and flight. Several meetings have to be dedicated to explore the known and the unknown causes that "depotentiate" the client's immune system. So far we know that in most cases, cancer is the corollary of many years of tragedy. This is why it is of primary importance to explore these events, to put them forth for the client to reprocess them.

It is also important for client and practitioner to know why this cancer was produced and how the client unconsciously influenced immunomodulation to produce this onset. It is of primary importance to explore what purpose this cancer serves.

A cancer patient is also a depressed person; therefore, we have to accommodate this depression in the treatment plan.

The difference between this approach to healing and a typical treatment for depression is that we have to mobilize not only mechanisms for emotional healing, but also mechanisms for physical healing.

It is important for the practitioner to know that the most difficult part of the treatment is the sale to the client of the idea that healing is possible. This is the idea that has to be discussed with the physician as a doable scenario. As sometimes happens, practitioners are not keen in providing "false hopes"— which, in my book, is an oxymoron. Like any sale, you have to start from the end. That is, the practitioner should assume that the client is capable of successfully attaining the goal of surviving.

Patient and practitioner have to know the direction of the treatment; it is of maximal importance to create a road map containing the focus and direction of it. This treatment needs to include a timeframe within which the goals are to be achieved.

In my practice, when in contact with physicians, I recognize that this medical practitioner is performing a difficult balancing act. Firstly, the society has endowed him with power and a mandate that demands dedication and responsibility. The society gave him a position of power, turned him into somebody whose words and opinions have an extraordinary weight. This professional does not want to risk an opinion that might jeopardize his position as a sage (or face a lawsuit from a patient that is using this opinion as a weapon against this professional). Everything has to be scientifically sound. The problem is . . . How scientifically sound can hope be?

Is there a laboratory instrument to measure commitment and resilience?

This stance makes him sometimes unable to provide the hopes and assurances the client needs to hear.

The Edmonton Journal of May 21, 2007, in an article named "Medicine without Borders" profiled two physicians with opposing views on medicine. Dr. Mark Sherman (a young physician from

Victoria, B.C.) stated "I feel very strongly that an integrative approach to health, including the whole environment and the whole person, is an inevitable evolution in health care." Meanwhile, Dr. Lloyd Oppel (the spokesman from the B.C. Medical Association) stated "Just because people have genuine credentials, it doesn't mean that everything they have to say is scientifically supportable. It can really give the gloss of a lot of scientific validity to a conference [with regard to the Body Heals Conference from May 25 to 27, 2007) . . . With scientific medicine taken for granted, it's not surprising that people wanting more are turning to imaginative sources for health."

I believe this controversy is still on.

Achieving Rapport

Rapport as a Lower-Left Quadrant Activity

The Lower Left Quadrant (LL) contains the experience of the collective, such as culture and relationships. It is the "WE," the subjective side of the relationship.

This is the quadrant containing the relationship between client and therapist.

Successful interactions depend on our ability to establish and maintain rapport. Surprisingly, we make most decisions based on rapport rather than on technical merits; for I more likely trust, agree with, or support someone I can relate to.

Rapport is conceptualized as a relationship marked by harmony, conformity, accord, or affinity. It supports agreement, alignment, likeness, or similarity. Establishing rapport is creating an instant positive first impression, and once rapport is achieved, the client can be led into a pre-trance state.

Rapport involves being in alignment with another individual, matching body language, matching vocabular universe, and accepting and utilizing the individual's reality. Standing or sitting in an identical position with the client is a way to start achieving rapport. Physical matching has to be achieved as naturally as possible, making a feedback loop that would provide the client with ample opportunities to relax. Voice adjustment, matching gestures, and facial expressions are to be used from the very first minute in which the encounter between therapist and client is produced. Lead systems—visual, auditory, or kinesthetic—must be used to present ideas in the way preferred by the client.

Constantly calibrating the client and reading his/her external observable behaviors will provide the therapist with basic information on the client's internal state. One of such internal states is the hostility that sometimes is demonstrated by the so-called resistant client. By recognizing the existence of these behaviors and by legitimizing the right of the client to observe and act upon these behaviors, the therapist places himself in a position to utilize these behaviors to create rapport.

All behaviors exhibited by the client represent an opportunity to communicate effectively. Instead of concentrating on where the client is coming from, we can introduce a positive frame by concentrating on where the client is going. From here onward, we take the client into the future.

In order to pace and lead all behaviors, we need to have the acuity or sensitivity to notice whether or not we are producing a positive impact on the client. Acuity will allow us to observe if what we are doing is working; our flexibility (a very important quality the therapist must have) will allow us to change course and make adjustments to the therapeutic process.

Pacing the client outside his conscious awareness allows us to facilitate unconscious generative processes. It is important to remember that our unconscious mind is the more aware and the wiser of the two minds. Even though we need to establish rapport to induce trance, hypnosis also facilitates and increases rapport. During trance the client's attention is turned inward, and the operator/therapist becomes his only contact with the external reality. His attention is focused only on the therapist's voice, which can direct the client's attention toward achieving therapeutic goals. This is rapport at its best.

Gathering Information

Each client is a universe. There is no one like him; therefore, there must be no assumptions or prejudgments in the analysis of his life experiences.

Type and quality of the gathered information is of utmost importance. On that account, I am isolating two elements that, in my opinion, fulfill this requisite. These elements are:

2.1. The clinician must be prepared, emotionally and intellectually, to understand the client's life experience.

2.2. The client has to be able to comprehend the concepts used by the practitioner when the practitioner is translating ("trance-lating") client's experiences into a treatment plan.

This might sound very elemental, but the reader would be surprised to know the percentage of treatments that fail just because the verbal and nonverbal dialogue was never established during the first meeting.

A client may feel uncomfortable if a practitioner does not focus on the problem immediately. He must be certain that he is getting involved in a therapeutic process rather than in a social situation. If small talk predominates, he may think that the therapist is not interested in his problem.

The client should come out of the first meeting with the impression that something good has happened and that something was achieved.

An important goal of the first stage of information gathering is to obtain clear and detailed descriptions of problems and experiences as perceived by the client, and to become familiar with their linguistic patterns and generative themes. This will allow the practitioner to recognize the client's patterns and idiosyncratic mode of organization of internal experiences.

This is the stage in which the overall goal is to create a context for action and meaningful changes. Through questioning and leading comments, the therapist begins orientating the client toward *creating a representation of a reality consonant with the treatment*; in this case, orientating the client toward the future.

Through asking questions, we lead the client toward a transformation of his perception of reality.

There is nothing wrong in asking leading questions if the objective is to guide the client toward pattern-interruption or symptom-interruption.

The first premise in this process is that by orientating the client toward the future, we will be able to create expectations for therapeutic changes.

The second premise is that each problem is carrying its solution within. This is the basis for transformational change. The change must be produced inside out (i.e. it must come from within).

When asking questions and making meaningful and leading comments, it is important to use the same vocabular universe and linguistic structure that the client is using to define the problem. The solution must be consonant with these two elements. Problem and solution should be explained using the same types of words. Questioning should be directed toward a confirmation of the client's sense of social identity. Instead of a dry interrogation on personal statistics (such as birthdate, social insurance number, etc.), we should use the opportunity to ascertain their social values. Questions should be asked regarding family structure, family relationship, goals and hopes, children, peer groups, religious orientation, etc. This information will provide the therapist with an overview of the client's perception of his social reality and social context.

Throughout the conversations (avoid interrogating the client), the therapist should reinforce the uniqueness of the client as a person. We need to remember that this is the stage in which instillation of hope takes place, thereby, motivating the client to enter into a therapeutic alliance. The client has to think that in this meeting, he has acquired something of value. He should come out of the meeting feeling that his time and money were well spent and the meeting was worthwhile.

Instillation of Hope or Building Expectancy

I made a habit to accompany my wife to most of her medical appointments. I would like to remind the reader that we were living in Northern Alberta, Canada—where distances and travel conditions are measured in hours of travelling instead of kilometers, and weather advisory is consulted prior to travelling. Awareness of road condition is a must to avoid unpleasant experiences.

On one occasion when my wife had an appointment with a mental health practitioner, she came out of the meeting feeling more depressed than she was at the beginning of the appointment. I had to use the return trip travel time (five hours) to absorb all the anger and the frustration projected by my wife as the result of an unproductive meeting with an uninterested practitioner, wherein a healing goal was not achieved. It was a good thing that we both are mental health practitioners and are, therefore, prepared for this kind of situation.

Can you imagine this happening to a couple less prepared to confront the aftermath of a psychiatric interview? I wondered on that occasion about how many couples divorced after a psychiatric exploration.

This psychiatrist forgot that an interview is like a surgical procedure. We open the patient to do exploratory emotional surgery, and at the end of the process, we have to close the wound; otherwise, this patient will emotionally bleed to death.

As a consequence of leaving the emotional wound open, we expose the client to develop fear networks that might compromise the achievement of therapeutic goals. At the end of every session, we must create some form of closure.

We open the client's emotional wound at the beginning of the meeting and suture the wound at the end of the procedure.

A cancer patient is generally a depressed patient with negative expectations of his future. Fear, depression, self-pity, and rage are altering his delicate mental and emotional balance. This client discerns that something is out of control and subsequently feels powerless in his battle against this monster that is growing inside his bodymind.

Since he feels that his body is an out-of-control enemy, it is absolutely necessary to provide him with the hope that there are many things that are still within his control. This is the precise slice of time in which the skills of the therapist should be employed to create in the client a sense of control of what is happening in his life. The client has to learn that he/she has capabilities within his/her bodymind to alter the progress of the sickness.

In order for the patient to internalize the idea that the future holds promises of recovery, basic techniques for control should be demonstrated.

My best demonstration tool is the hypnotic alteration of perceptions of pain.

I utilize the client's experience of pain to demonstrate practically that he has access to some systems/techniques that can provide relief from fear and pain. One technique that I frequently use—and the most enticing to the client—is local anesthesia using glove anesthesia.

I noticed that, in the case of cancer patients, they need compelling evidence of the power of their unconscious mind, as well as proof of the existence of mind-body tools for recovery. Convincers are important. Amnesia, symptom substitution, hypnotic confusion, and relocation of pain are excellent convincers; for they provide immediate symptomatic relief.

It is important to add that cancer patients experiencing pain are already in a light trance state; therefore, it is relatively easy to induce a deeper trance.

UPPER RIGHT QUADRANT (UR)

	Upper Right (UR) INDIVIDUAL "IT" Body and Behaviors Procedures

The Upper Right quadrant identifies the procedures, actions, and personal competencies of the therapist, as well as client's competencies that can be utilized in the treatment. It is where the treatment plan takes form.

Integrity and Hypnotherapy

Integrity can be conceptualized as the degree of consistency and interdependence existing between the parties associated with the healing process.

Full support for the patient's quest for change, the setting aside of personal bias, the acceptance of individual experiences as valid and true, and the avoidance of prescription-like solutions are at the base of integral clinical hypnotherapeutic experiences. As a professional in the field, I am aware that there is an element of power in the commanding of the communication to persuade the client to make changes in his/her mental maps. Every effort is placed on the enhancement of individual capabilities to produce meaningful changes. After all, therapy is conceptualized as the art of using communication to facilitate in the client a flow of creating expression.

Stephen Gilligan, an Ericksonian Hypnotherapist, mentions that an effective hypnotic communicator produces a state of controlled spontaneity. In this state, the parties never know what they are going to do next because they adhere to a set of general guidelines to provide effectiveness and complex flexibility to the process. He also mentions several principles that govern the Ericksonian Therapy Model in which the value of integrity is primary.

> Integrity is the degree by which the therapist's intentions and expressions are aligned with the needs of the client . . . Integrity is the context from which all self-valuing expressions are generated. (Gilligan 1987, p. 64)

Integrity involves walking the same path the client does and actively listening to every utterance that could provide an insight into his world. This stance allows the therapist to visualize the client's world as close as possible—prior to immersing into the client's experience, protecting and accepting his view of the world, pacing him and leading him into achieving meaningful change.

Integrity is what is at the base of the Cooperation Principle in Ericksonian Hypnotherapy.

Developing and Maintaining Integrity

Stephen Gilligan recognizes three options to achieve and maintain integrity.

1. Identification and handling of unacceptable personal experiences

Personal attachments (fears, problems, etc.), biased perceptions, rigidity, and lack of acceptance of others place a limit in what a therapist can achieve.

While working with Louise, I had to deal with my own limitations, my third-world experiences and biases, especially the ones originated on personal views and values coming from experiences with the culture of poverty in South American First Nations.

Oftentimes it is difficult to self-identify and consciously recognize deeply personal, unacceptable experiences. It is very difficult to be mindful of biases that might block the resolve of our client to talk about their unique experiences. I might tend to judge an experience as unacceptable because I am filtering this client's experience through the filter of my own very personal biases. Here lies the importance of the Utilization Principle as a tool to align our experiences with client's experiences to facilitate change and healing with integrity.

2. Be non-evaluative.

It is suggested that the therapist should refrain from classifying the client in diagnostic categories. This principle brings to mind the issue of diagnostic tools widely used by mental health practitioners such as the Diagnostic and Statistical Manual of Mental Disorders (DSM-IV-TR), which is produced by the American Psychiatric Association. This manual enables the practitioner to label the client as suffering a specific illness based on pre-classified symptoms. It brings to mind the case of a child "belonging" to the Government of Alberta's foster care system, which blamed all his alleged inabilities, behaviors, and academic performance on his diagnostic of being a "Fetal Alcohol Syndrome "child. I am wondering whether the practitioner diagnosed or labeled this child.

3. Facilitating space for clients to generate their own experiences.

The command of the communication enables the practitioner to have a measure of power over the client, which may inadvertently give the practitioner the opportunity to violate his integrity. A therapist that is mindful of the rights of the client will increase his/her client's chances to succeed in producing meaningful changes. The opposite option will bring only frustration and disappointment to a practitioner that considers himself responsible for the client's experience.

The role of the therapist is to stimulate and motivate the client into action, the content of the action being the full responsibility of the client.

We have to praise our client's mind for knowing what she wants . . . consciously . . . and unconsciously . . . (because) your unconscious mind already knows what is needed to achieve what has to be achieved . . . and you already made up your mind about how . . . and when . . . this is going to happen . . . surely knowing the outcome . . . a positive outcome already planned by your unconscious mind . . . since it already took a decision . . . a firm decision of what is good for you and . . . what and when you will start . . . to do what has to be done . . . since you already decided to go ahead . . . and do it . . .

During the sessions, I try to be as meaningfully vague as possible, attempting to reverse pathological thoughts by using metaphors such as . . . I had a magnet once . . . that I used to find all the good things made out of metal that I could use again . . . to solve a problem . . . whatever I lost . . . nails, screws, pieces of rebar . . . connectors . . . I found them again to keep on building my project . . . whatever I wanted to find . . . I found with my magnet . . .

Being meaningfully vague allows the client to utilize his own unconscious experiences instead of me imposing some of my own biases.

Trancework Preparation: Changework and Alteration of Physical and Emotional Experiences

In this stage, we assume that the client has already accepted the notion of the bodymind as possessing tools to produce healing. Here they will be introduced to different stages of relaxation and visualization/imagery.

This is the stage in which the accumulated information acquired in the first meeting is "trance-formed" into visualizations for deep relaxation and changework. Training of the patient in inducing relaxation and a trance state is obtained through progressive approximations toward trance, such as the Refractionation Method (in which the client is briefly trance-induced several times, each time longer and in a deeper level of trance) and the Modeling Trance (in which the therapist gives to the client a demonstration of self-induced trance).

In this stage, it is assumed that the client has already accepted the therapeutic contract and that he is already in a light trance, the product of an appropriate creation of expectations toward the future. We also reassure the client that through a strong commitment to the program, attaining relief and remission of their sickness is a possibility

Many times we hear the cautionary message: "Don't induce false hopes to the patient." This message is typically a product of the fear of a practitioner to be confronted with failure. To this practitioner, it is safer to tell the clients that his life is terminally threatened by a sickness than to suggest that there is a possibility of recovery. If the patient dies, the practitioner demonstrated that his prognosis was correct. If the person recovers, it is going to be the product of the excellent care performed by the practitioner.

In no one moment was this practitioner at risk. The only person that was at risk was the patient.

After an iatrogenic comment, the odds are against the patient. A timid and insecure practitioner will instill in the client more doubts than certainties in recovering his health.

This is the risk that the practitioner has to take. It is a leap of faith. This is also the reason why I do not work on palliative care as my primary concern. Even if I agree that palliative care has an important place in the care of the chronically ill patients, I am also of the belief that palliative care should be provided when the patient is truly ready for it and when it is the only alternative left to them.

Experience tells me that successful patients were never the pessimistic or the giving-up types; rather, they were risk-takers with a strong belief in what they were attempting to achieve.

The therapeutic contract must include from the patient and the practitioner a firm commitment toward recovery. For that reason, it is an important part of preparation work.

Changework and Mind Regulation

Elliott Dacher, MD, suggests that the mind, if left to itself, will recall and repeat what it has learned however false and destructive may the recalled content be, rather than remembering its natural gifts. He adds that it is possible to break through the barriers of brain biology and learned ignorance, replacing misconceived contents with authentic, personal, and enriching knowledge through Mindfulness Techniques, as well as through the use of a habit-forming mechanism he calls Conscious Living. The objective is to unlearn misperceptions that are forcing us to develop behaviors inconsistent with our health. (Dacher 1991,pp. 154–155)

Conscious Living uses the innate capacities of the mind to establish new habits by exposing ourselves to repetitive new behaviors. The purpose of this exercise is to reprogram our minds in accordance with our new and different perceptions, subsequently creating a healthy life and a healthy lifestyle. Subsequently this will create the context in which we will regulate and change the most intractable and unhealthy aspect of our Mind-Talk.

Mind-talk, as the predominant function of the mind, is the result of the interaction of our sensory systems and the social environment.

Even if we are not yet prepared for change, we can act *as if* we had already integrated these new learnings. An example of healthy conscious living is the balance obtained when we avoid extreme behaviors, observing instead a lifestyle that keeps an adequate proportion of time spent in outer activities and personal, private space (solitude).

Unhealthy mind-talk includes powerlessness—which is translated into helplessness, inadequacy, and loneliness, which is experienced as isolation and deprivation. Mind-talk produced during these states is responsible for emotional distress, fear, worry, and anxiety.

Dr. Dacher explains that healing starts in the mind at the precise moment when we decide to take charge of our illness. Since birth, as we grow, we accumulate an increasingly large file of experiences, memories, and stored information that stimulate the main activity of our mind, which is translated as mind-talk. At the same time that our mind accumulates negative experiences, it also assembles capabilities for mindfulness, attention, concentration, and meditation that we rarely use. We express Mind-talk through thoughts, images, sensations, and feelings, creating in turn behaviors and attitudes which guide our lifestyle. This mixture of healthy and unhealthy attitudes could move us toward emotional balance and health, as well as toward emotional stress, physiological stress, and disease.

Throughout our lives, we gravitate toward health; but we are also pulled toward disease.

One of the notions at the base of Dr. Dacher's philosophy is Mindfulness, this notion also being the centerpiece of Dr. Jon Kabat-Zinn's work (which he describes in his book Full Catastrophe Living). Mindfulness and Mind-talk, both concepts shared by Dr. Dacher, are the two main activities of the operating systems of the mind. I would like to concentrate on these two concepts—which, in my opinion, are directly related to trance and trancework, as well as to the concept of self-regulation or self-modulation of the bodymind.

Both concepts are part—or should be part—of the conventional medical treatment, diagnostic, and therapy.

Mindfulness and self-regulation are directed toward promoting health and primary prevention. Mindfulness and mind-talk, as operating systems of the mind cannot, in Dr. Dacher's opinion, operate simultaneously. I am of the opinion that the author errs in believing this assumption to be true.

While mind-talk is conceptualized as the predominantly automatic mental chatter, mindfulness is a self-initiated activity of the mind; and it requires conscious efforts to be produced.

Mind

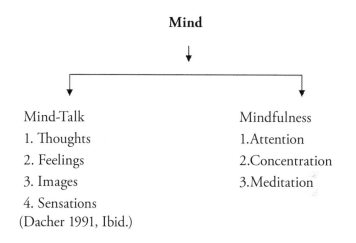

Mind-Talk
1. Thoughts
2. Feelings
3. Images
4. Sensations
(Dacher 1991, Ibid.)

Mindfulness
1. Attention
2. Concentration
3. Meditation

The four aspects of mind-talk might be activated at any time. Mindfulness's aspects occur sequentially: Attention is followed by concentration, which precedes meditation. Mind-talk relies on stored information, which in the author's opinion is always a recollection from the past, from experiences stored in the memory files. This information is divided into two categories: Factual information and Psychological information.

Factual information provides us with access to knowledge about places and objects. Recalling factual information is, in the opinion of the author, usually but not always useful. It allows us to work more efficiently, making correct decisions, and automatically allowing us to use sophisticated technical devices.

Without mindfulness, factual information can be quite destructive (i.e. using nuclear power to develop weapons, or polluting our environment).

Psychological information can be healthy or unhealthy, the unhealthy information inaccurate and false being. Healthy psychological information comes from life experiences that support healthy emotional development. It causes neither pain nor suffering; and it leads to the development of healthy attitudes, actions, and lifestyles. This information, factual and psychological, can remain dormant and be recalled through events and circumstances that unlock our memory.

I think that, even though the author's opinions are very valuable to understand the way mindfulness and mind-talk functions, some of his assumptions deserve some reflection.

He states that mindfulness and mind-talk cannot operate simultaneously. I posit that the contrary happens and every chunk of experience and information is unconsciously stored in our data bank through a permanent, uninterrupted process of automatic information gathering.

While the mind is processing factual, conscious information during awareness, our unconscious mind is simultaneously gathering and storing information in our unconscious mind, which the author correctly assumes is our memory bank. Also, the author creates a dichotomy between mind-talk and mindfulness, one being automatic (unconscious?) and the other occurring in total awareness.

Recent research suggests that both operating systems act in conscious and unconscious levels simultaneously. Studies on the unconscious function of the mind (adaptive unconscious) suggests that while our conscious mind is occupied we can perform quick, non-conscious analysis and evaluate and select information that suits our purposes (Wilson, T. 2002, p. 15-16)

Changework and Communication

Perception of Reality

A while ago I was invited to attend a conference at the Faculty of Education of the University of Alberta in Edmonton, Alberta, Canada. The topic was "Communication and Education: A comparative analysis of the philosophy of Gramsci and Paulo Freire." A friend of mine, a professor in the same faculty knew of my prior training in the pedagogy of Paulo Freire, as well as of my experiences in the use of Freire's methods during my tenure as professor at the University of Chile. One of the subjects discussed was transformational communication and the problem of social alienation.

As the subject was introduced, I was confronted with the dilemma of the mechanicism in the communication; how communication can become a simply ineffective tool of transmission of information. I learned that there is more to communication than a dialogue and a casual conversation. Communication exceeds the simple act of talking and, involved in this uniquely human act of uttering a word, were moral, ethical, and political elements qualifying and validating the act of emitting a message. The Moral Theories of Language of Jürgen Habermas and Emmanuel Levinas were analysed, starting with Levinas's reflections on the moral relevance of language, with a particular use of language as a conversation. He stated . . . "The very fact of being in a conversation consists in recognizing in the other a right over one's egoism, and hence in justifying oneself" (Hendley, 1956). It made me think of the many programs I watched in my life in where the presenter was so much in love with his own voice and with his own self that he did not notice that the audience was already gone somewhere, to a better mentally and emotionally place.

The "face of the other," which Levinas evokes as the ground of the human being's sense of moral obligation, is essentially the face of my interlocutor, my client which is addressing me in speech. My client is the "other" that qualifies my message. There lies the moral obligation to make my speech meaningful to him, who in turn will reward me by validating my existence.

The meaning of the communication is established in the conversation as the interlocutor . . . "is called upon to speak" . . . and in so doing comes to the assistance of their word. Herein lays the essentially magisterial character of speech; the way which my interlocutor presents himself as interlocutor, as irreducible to anything said insofar as he maintains the right to say more, to comment on what is said.

To this extent, my interlocutor is my master, my teacher, my client, the one to whom I am obliged to be attentive" (Hendley, 1956).

In a way, I see a parallel between the interlocutor, a person who reads or judges the written statement of the author and reacts accordingly to the content, and the client who is my interlocutor, and gives meaning to my effort to help him in transforming his (and mine) reality. I owe to my clients to be their therapist in the same way that the author is given meaning by the simple act of somebody reading his book. Any person involved in a communication in which the interlocutor is the recipient of the message, is therefore qualified and justified by the communication.

To the therapist, this point in which communication takes place is important in the way that speech is understood only when is made acceptable, when the content of the speech gives origin to an action.

If fairness of communication involves our concern for others, describing contents of the communication implies also an account of our own perceptions of what we are communicating.

I am wondering how many times during a meeting I assumed that I knew what my client needed; because I simply did not listen to him, I just assumed that what I had in mind was exactly what he needed from me.

No wonder he/she never came back to see me again.

As a therapist, we constantly err by assuming we can read our client's mind.

Because we do not see the world as it is, rather interpreting the world based on our own perceptions, the question of integrity becomes paramount.

As I stated in previous chapters, integrity is important when dealing with somebody's emotional contents.

Can a person act with integrity outside of these perceptions?

The truth is nobody can.

Perception and credibility are basic tenets of communication. While perception directs behavior using as a guide a personal interpretation of an experience or situation, credibility is manifested in the form of one interlocutor questioning the sincerity, integrity, and competence of the other. Credibility problems give way to communication breakdowns.

Every therapist is aware that in order to establish rapport, the client has to trust his judgment. Perception problems, on the other hand, are easy to solve once the individual realizes that what he sees is not what it is, but rather it is their way to interpret their sensorial perception. Perception, on the other hand, can easily create self-fulfilling prophecies.

There are many immune-suppressive illnesses that result from self-fulfilling prophecies.

Perception is projection, is an important law of communication. The reality that I perceive is only my perception, not necessarily what my client perceives or should perceive. Reality is just a personal opinion. As a therapist, I owe to my clients to accept that what they perceive is the truth, "their" truth; therefore, we have to work with their perceptions, legitimizing it first, and then discussing its validity. This is one of the most valuable tenets of the Utilization Principle in Ericksonian Hypnotherapy.

I am fortunate to have a spouse that is very competent in keeping my feet solidly anchored to the ground, to a reality that provides me with a much needed balance to properly grasp an experience, reflect on it, and extract conclusions that are valid to me and to my interlocutor.

A while ago, with great ingenuity, she pointed out that, in order to introduce a therapeutic thought, every situation has to be analyzed in the here-and-now. She illustrated her position with the following metaphor:

"A while ago, a man was living in California. He lived like any person in this California weather, perfectly adapted to his environment.

Suddenly, like in a dream, he found himself wandering in a town near the Arctic Circle. For the first time, he experienced the chill of the arctic wind penetrating his skin, permeating the California clothing he was still wearing. In desperation, he searched for anything that he could use to cover himself, to defend himself from this cold arctic wind for which he was utterly unprepared. He found some straw, discarded plastic, and used fabric and made himself a coat to keep warm and to survive. He endured suffering and desperation, but his coat kept him alive.

One day he received the notice that he was going back to California.

The first thing he put in his luggage was his coat made of discarded straw, plastic, and fabric."

Why did this person, who knew the difference of temperature between California and the Arctic, placed such high value on this coat and kept it, when he was informed that he was going home?

Many interpretations can be extracted from this tale.

When in danger, we resort to any mechanism to survive, which we consider suitable for a particular situation. When our circumstances change, it is difficult to let go of these survival mechanisms that sustained us in difficult times. It seems it is in our human nature to be afraid of letting go of something that was useful in a troubling situation.

Oftentimes, it is hard to discern whether the survival mechanisms we resorted to survive and adapt in the past, are still suitable for the present situation. Our emotional attachment to these mechanisms sometimes block our capacity to discriminate about what part is still useful in the here-and-now, and what part can or should be discarded. As mentioned in prior chapter, we customarily "transcend and include" some parts of our experiences from the past, even the ones that are no longer needed.

In order to overcome pathological experiences from the past, we need to "transcend" them, to go beyond these experiences into a different level of being, in a continual spiral. Some of these experiences will be discarded, and some parts will be "included" in the new level of existence as learnings. Wisdom is attained in a repeated spiral of learning, for life does not evolve horizontally, but vertically; each level of existence leading us toward the future, the spiral changing from a Present Way of Being (PWOB) to a New Way of Being (NWOB) (Divine L. 2009,p. 62)

Sometimes we get stuck in the present, and like the aforementioned traveller, keep something no longer useful, just because it is comfortable and familiar.

In situations of this nature, the role of the therapist becomes paramount in helping the client to discriminate between maladaptive behaviours they are using in this here-and-now, and adaptive, constructive behaviors.

It would be advisable for the therapist and the client to dedicate a segment of the session or sessions to analyse whether the client is using mechanisms to *survive,* and when and how this *surviving* would change into *living.*

We have to keep in mind that clients have the capability to take their own decisions, and if sometimes they feel unable to proceed, it might be due to their bodymind being unable to discriminate between a healthy behavior and a pathological behavior . . . which brings to the fore another problem:

What can be considered a healthy behavior?

This question should be answered using sociocultural and psychological parameters.

There are cultural determinants that establish what is healthy as a synonym of what is socially accepted; what is sane for the individual as well as for the society.

In Canada, we are living in a cultural mosaic that sometimes challenges the therapist to adapt to almost impossible situations. In some places, children could wear long braids in the Canadian aboriginal way, a kirpan (a mostly ceremonial dagger used by some members of the Sikh community), a hijab (a fabric that covers a girl's head) or a turban.

These determinants mostly demonstrate that the answer about what is accepted as a healthy behavior is not in the hands of the therapist, but in the client's decision to determine what is acceptable.

No wonder Erickson and Zeig thought that the essence of psychotherapy was about "reframing," clearly establishing the difference between "therapy" and "counselling" or the giving of advice. They believe (and I believe) that therapy is all about reframing, which they conceptualized as "changing the perceived meaning of something" (Zeig, J. 1994, pp. 212-215)

This is a situation that merits further discussion.

PART V

MEDICAL HYPNOSIS: A TRUE ORGANIC APPROACH

LOWER RIGHT QUADRANT

	LOWER RIGHT (LR) **COLLECTIVE "ITS"** **Structures and Systems**

The Lower Right quadrant represents what we do, the way we implement the treatment plan, the structures that are involved in the process, such as hospitals, clinics, organizations, legal systems regulating service delivery, as well as the systems that are monitoring the effectiveness of the plan. It globally represents the structures and systems connected with the client and the practitioner.

What is Medical Hypnosis?

Medical Hypnosis is conceptualized as a special type of interchange between two people, in which trance is involved and utilized to accomplish a therapeutically valuable result. Medical hypnosis is cost effective and, in the opinion of many therapists, me included, produces quick results.

Many books have been written on the subject of the history of trance and its evolution. I would like, for the sake of space and time, to refer the reader to the many excellent books written on the subject of hypnosis.

We already know that the power of hypnosis resides in the patient, who might indicate that any hypnosis is self-hypnosis. There is ample research that proves that patients undergoing hypnosis do better during medical procedures, recovering from them or ameliorating or surmounting side effects of treatment when they are relaxed and hopeful.

Medical hypnosis and clinical hypnotherapy are one and the same. Both demand the use of the patient's experiences to achieve healing. Both put the patient at the centre of the attention. Medical hypnosis adds more tools to the arsenal of modern medicine, which historically tends to minimize the existence or importance of autonomous therapeutic processes, relying solely on conscious and voluntary experiences. It adds to the process the unconscious dimension of individual experiences, as well as the understanding of automatic and involuntary processes that are controlled by the unconscious mind.

Medical hypnosis recognizes the capabilities of the patient to use the full potential of his state–dependent information, as well as accepting that certain aspects of organic diseases are connected to involuntary neural or neurochemical control systems.

Today, we know that hypnosis can potentiate the healing of a variety of psychological and physical problems. Symptoms are "signals" produced by the bodymind for the practitioner to decode and utilize to facilitate healing.

As early as 1840, Dr. James Esdaile, in India, developed hypnotherapeutic methods as coadjutant in surgery. Dr. Esdaile used hypnotic trance as an effective anaesthetic before chemical anaesthesia was even created.

As of today, many physicians are endorsing the use of imagery and visualization as part of medical procedures; distress-relieving procedures introduced before and after surgical procedures, are some of the present uses of hypnosis in a medical setting. About a month ago, my wife underwent surgery to repair a rotator cuff. As it is customary in Canadian hospitals, she was summoned to the Grey Nuns Hospital in Edmonton, Alberta, for an interview with all the professionals that were going to be involved in the procedure. She had an interview with an anaesthesiologist, a physiotherapist, and an orthopaedic surgeon.

Among the instructions, she was given a CD containing a relaxation exercise and visualization to be used prior to surgery, and another one to be used after surgery. My first thought was that, finally, health systems were acknowledging the value of conscious–unconscious preparedness for surgery and healing.

Hypnosis and the Treatment of Cancer

Despite all the research and technological advances, cancer remains one of the main causes of death. We have already detailed all the circumstances associated with the cancer sufferer. Patients diagnosed with cancer confront a deep multilevel crisis associated with anxiety and fear of death, and physical and emotional pain connected with chemotherapy, radiation therapy, and with invasive surgical procedures taking its toll in their immune system.

Cancer affects the individual from the cellular level to the psychological level. To ameliorate this multilevel crisis, I utilize hypnotic trance to produce a significant impact on the outcome of the disease. It is my belief that trance is instrumental in the treatment of immunodeficient sicknesses like cancer.

As early as 1966, Arnold M. Ludwig mentioned that beneath a veneer of consciousness lies an uncharted territory which corresponds to the altered states of consciousness, which are mental estates induced by physiological, psychological or pharmacological manoeuvring producing a distortion in subjective experience or psychological functioning (Ludwig. A., as mentioned in Tart, C. "Altered States of Consciousness", 1969).

The individual acknowledges this state subjectively, and this distortion may be manifested when a person discovers a lump in a breast or an unidentified growth in an area of the body. As a result, negative self-hypnosis, an alteration of the normal, customary state of mentation is produced. Negative emotions in the form of fear networks ensue, and a chain reaction is produced by the combination of basic emotions altering the otherwise normal mental state of the individual. Corresponding imagery will permeate every though in this suffering individual. We just cannot avoid creating images of everything that cross our mind, for we normally visualize our world through images.

A diagnosis of cancer produces an associated chain of emotions connected with feelings of sadness, disgust, anger and surprise, which mixed with secondary emotions, destabilizes the immune system. The individual becomes highly vulnerable to negative statements, which in turn may be interpreted by the unconscious mind as predictions of negative outcomes, i.e., a "you'll have to live with this pain" statement may be interpreted by our unconscious mind as a death sentence should the pain go away. If I do not feel the pain, my very factual unconscious mind might conclude that I am dying. (Tart, C. 1969, p. 11); (Themes, R. 1999, pgs. 107-108).

A caregiver should be aware that nonverbal and verbal communications are vehicles for wellness as well as for a departure from wellness. Caregivers become endowed with the responsibility of reframing these perceptions; therefore it is imperative for them to receive training in the basic tenets of medical hypnosis and communication.

Since patients are utilizing positive and negative preconceptions, every therapeutic intervention should start with an intake in which the practitioner will gather comprehensive information about the magnitude of the disease. This information will allow the practitioner to help the client control and eliminate misconceptions, and reframe perceptions created with the little information he is usually given.

The therapist has to bear in mind that an uncertain client may create a devastating picture of his illness. Hypnosis can be therefore instrumental in transforming negative perceptions that might be blocking attempts to reverse the sickness.

Hypnosis can be instrumental in working with the symptoms, pain amelioration and nonspecific symptoms such as fatigue and emotional distress. It has been helpful in the management of side effects, in providing psychological adjustment of the client to his social milieu and, most important, instrumental in modifying immune response to alter the course of a disease.

Clarification of timelines[19] and instillation of hope for a positive (and real) outcome should be considered paramount in any treatment. Reference material such as books and other information should be left with the patient to reinforce the importance of actively participating in the healing process. It is advisable for the patient to also receive training in self-hypnosis.

In the same way that symptoms are experienced in a unique way from individual to individual, treatment should be tailored to fit the very idiosyncratic needs of the client.

The goals of treatment can be summarised as follows:

- **Reassertion of ego strength to face the crisis**
Therapy should primarily concentrate on instillation of hope and ego support, via providing the client with tools for self-empowerment to meet crisis, such as techniques for self-hypnosis, meditation, imagery and visualizations for recovery. One of the benefits of meditation is the information that is acquired through self-examination of internal forces, energy, emotions, and the empowerment that this knowledge generates.

---

[19] A timeline is a way to display life events in a chronological order. I use timelines to organize events leading to a sickness. (Author's note)

Each individual reacts in a very personalized and idiosyncratic way to an intervention, in the same way that the same medication produces different reactions in different individuals. The uniqueness of the individual cannot be ignored.

Since healing is also a problem solving process, most of the responsibility is in the client's hand. The therapist acts as a facilitator of empowerment techniques to attain recovery.

- **Relief of Physical and Emotional Pain and of the resulting Fear and Anxiety**

Hypnosis can be used to modulate the presence of pain, altering and neutralizing the perception of painful stimuli. The experience of pain can be altered by the use of glove anaesthesia and inductions for pain control, displacement of the painful focus from one place to another or, if possible, removing pain altogether.

When the experience of pain is modified, the client is free to concentrate on reactivating his immune system, through improving quality of life and enjoying a meaningful existence.

Pain and fear of pain consume a great deal of energy at the expense of recovery and healing.

During my work with Freesia, I felt blessed by the possibility of providing a safe place for her to feel protected, empowered, and ready to embark on the healing journey, which in her case lasted several years. I failed miserably when, ten years before Freesia, I tried to do the same with my wife Matilde.

She did not feel safe enough with me because she could perceive the fear produced by the lack of information, for at the time of her first cancer I was not a practitioner.

This experience taught me that as soon as we think of failure as a possibility, our resolve becomes compromised. Once compromised, we automatically create within ourselves a blueprint for failure.

While modern medicine has the use of many diagnostic devices, from X rays machines to MRI's, there is not a single device that replaces the human touch to create motivation for wellness. Conversely, it is practically impossible to measure results and progress without the diagnostic technology that modern medicine has at its disposal.

Specific therapeutic Interventions

Therapeutic hypnosis as a tool for healing has been accepted as a legitimate instrument to mobilize individual capabilities to access and set in motion the process of recovering from ill health. Imagery can set in motion the recovery from physical illnesses by allowing the client to visualize the problem, transforming these visualizations into new images that can be reframed into sub-images that are different from the original visualization. The mind, through the use of imagery, creates neural nets or neural programs to produce healing, not symptomatic relief, unless specifically requested, i.e., pain displacement and relocation.

Additionally, imagery produces changes in behavior by envisioning new possibilities.

Before implementing an intervention, we need to have a clear understanding of basic concepts. There is a difference between hypnotic induction and a hypnotic suggestion. While an *induction* is a standard and direct way to induce a hypnotic state, a *suggestion* is a comment that encourages people to believe in certain information.

Hypnosis is a normal, ordinary phenomenon that occurs every day, many times a day, and it is connected with our normal ultradian cycles[20]. It can be produced directly and indirectly, overtly or covertly, depending on what the practitioner wants to achieve and the decisions he wants to make to decide which would be the best way for a particular individual to access the trance state.

Anybody can produce a trance state; my favourite hypnotists are mothers who read bedtime stories to their children. When you

---

[20]   Ultradian cycles are a 90-to 120-minute basic rest-activity cycles responsible for the patterns of arousal, peak performance, stress and recovery that we experience every few hours. (Rossi, E.L. Ph.D. The 20-Minute Break. 1991)

observe these children totally absorbed and concentrated on the storyline, you will notice that they are in a trance state.

Throughout my work as a therapist, I have observed remarkable changes in individuals, changes that could have not happen in the waking state. I attempted, in most of my cases, to be nondirective, consciously ambiguous, maintaining the process as closed as possible to the particular experience of the client, utilizing his/her experiences to embed messages for change.

Every time I induce a trance, I am also driven into the same trance, becoming part of the same phenomenon, maintaining at the same time a certain detached position to retain control of the process. I learnt through practicing, that this is a common experience among practitioners, and a desirable experience to have, for it increases the rapport between practitioner and client. By maintaining an up-trance, I can communicate more effectively with my client.

The work of Milton Erickson, as well as the work of his disciples, has enabled me to add more techniques to my own repertoire.

My professional practice allows me to observe, adapt to, and adopt many tenets of different styles of therapeutic procedures. The work of Noam Chomsky initiated me in the analysis of how people communicate. I now look to select the proper language to create effective messages to meet specific needs, as well as where and how I am to be positioned to help my client to achieve meaningful changes.

My Guiding Therapeutic Principles

I spent many years researching, selecting and formulating guiding principles to work with my client's problems, learning in the process that I had to detach myself from any personal experience for it might create a bias in my professional judgment. I do not believe these principles are originals for I might have read them somewhere, perhaps in an occasion wherein I allowed my unconscious mind to harvest them from the therapy universe. I therefore apologize for my inability to mention their possible origin. From these experiences came my first principle.

Every departure from health is a family affair, in which every member also experience some form of departure from physical and emotional health.

I am aware of the difficulties involved in working with a member of my own family, but I had no other alternative. Like Erickson, who attempted to mitigate his own child's pain, I attempted to provide my spouse with opportunities for healing that, at that time, nobody else could dispense. People in pain, under normal circumstances, do not live disconnected from their milieu; therefore, the assessment of the client should also include their social context.

Every person connected with the client should learn to avoid catastrophic thoughts, learning in the process ways to deal with clients/patients that are catastrophizing.

My second principle reflects this reality.

The sufferer is experiencing pain, anguish and/or a paralyzing fear of their body and of their future.

Fear permeates every thought process, and mentation is altered, not allowing the person to think and plan adequately. Stress takes away hope and emotional balance.

My third principle states the following.

Every person in the sufferer's milieu has to become part of the therapeutic team. Every member should know a priori that any information or opinion conveyed to the sufferer would be incorporated unconsciously into the sufferer's mindset.

This principle came as a result of a visit from a particular religious sect that decided to start preparing the sufferer (my wife) to die within God's precepts. I had to expel them from our home, forbidding them to come back or to contact my wife. She did not want to die and her efforts were oriented toward regaining health. Also, a physician from the Grande Prairie Hospital commented to me that my wife's sickness was an irreversible process and that the cancer was going to spread to the bones; it was going to be a very painful and unstoppable outcome. He uttered not a single word about a possible positive outcome.

To avoid this situation, the fourth principle states the following. *Every communication produces changes in the sufferer's mental map; therefore, every communication must instil hope.* The sufferer is highly sensitive to the spoken language as well as to body languages. It is for this reason that the whole milieu has to be able to produce a congruent message for recovery.

The fifth principle states the following. *Any transformational work (Changework) has to address the sufferer's unconscious mind.* I am of the opinion that in order to be successful in transforming the mental model of the sufferer, we have to work with their unconscious mind to access their mental map. In the interest of producing deep and meaningful change, we need to access the deep structures of his mental model of communication, his state-dependent memory and learning, and state-bound behaviors. We need to remember that our most intelligent and informed mind is our unconscious mind.

Single stories are dangerous. The most common one is the story/perception associated with cancer as synonym of dying. Even today, people are still unwilling recipients of the single story of cancer associated with death, which overtly and covertly is all over the health system and the social milieu. In a meeting of a group of clients that were attending treatment in my office with a representative of the Faculty of Medicine of the University of Alberta in Edmonton, one of the clients complained about the memorial wall located at the entrance of the Cross Cancer Institute in Edmonton that, in her opinion was clearly telling the cancer sufferer that the logical next step is to die. The other side of the story, represented by the many successful recoveries, does not have the same exposure.

Pre-Trance Preparation

There is information available in the specialized literature that would allow the practitioner access to other practitioner's experiences and knowledge, avoiding in the process to "reinvent the wheel." Walters and Havens already compiled one of the most comprehensive lists of principles for pre-trance preparation. I used these principles intensively and I would like to incorporate them in this work, because they represent the way I envision trance.

I customarily start by attempting to create a mental picture of the individual that is coming to see me. Normally, I only know the way he/she sounded in the telephone interview, in which I took just basic information from this client. I prepare myself mentally and emotionally to produce an immediate rapport for I am aware that this person is in pain, and is coming to the meetings believing that I might be able to mitigate his pain. This is a big responsibility, therefore I mentally prepare myself to deliver what they hope to obtain.

His foray into my world has to be something they must enjoy.

In order to deliver the best service I am able to provide, I attempt to pursue very closely the following principles outlined by Walters and Havens.

1. *The client's well-being is my only concern.*

I am well aware that my role is to serve the client's purposes, not individual self-aggrandizement.

2. *The client decides what will happen and what will not.*

The client is in total control of his/her experience. I see myself as only the guide of his choice in his personal journey. I am in here to support him with the best of my abilities.

3. *The client must be protected at all times.*

This client's experience must be supported; his needs for comfort and safety are paramount. My primary role is to create a safe environment for my client to feel comfortable. I always include in the trance-scripts assurances that he will be protected and safe.

4. *The personal anxiety of the therapist has no place in a session.*

Prior to the session, I enter into a light self-hypnotic up-trance in which I convey to myself the following message . . . "I am well aware that my unconscious mind already knows what tools and skills are available to provide the services that my client demands. I am also aware that the knowledge and information that my client requires, will flow . . . little . . . by . . . little into my conscious mind, whenever I need these specific skills."

This is my way to prepare myself to be objective and to be in tune with my client's needs.

5. *A peaceful environment helps the client and the practitioner to achieve their objective.*

I am very fortunate to have the proper, comfortable setting for my client to relax. Any office that I used was close to a main street; therefore there were abundance of noises that I utilized in my inductions as . . . *"the sound of life around us."*

Since English is my second language, I have also incorporated in my inductions something that will eliminate my client's worries that he might not be able to understand my accent . . . *"and you may not know . . . consciously . . . what I am saying to you . . . but your unconscious mind will clearly understand the message I am conveying to your unconscious mind."*

Trancework: The Essence of Hypnotic Trance

There is an ample body of knowledge and relevant literature that can help the practitioner to create effective messages to address specific and nonspecific illnesses and emotional states. Ericksonian Hypnotherapy is a rich field from where we can extract general guidelines to create a trance state.

I am applying several principles of Ericksonian Hypnotherapy to create a frame from which I can write scripts that can be adapted to specific situations. I am mindful of the fact that a trance induction is not a standardized process. It requires observation and imagination, which is something that we all possess in abundance. Every induction is personal and uniquely crafted for the specific situation we are attempting to solve. Erickson and Rossi are insistent in that there are no universal methods for creating the same uniform trance state in every one undergoing a trance induction (Erickson M. and Rossi E. 1996. p. 3). In my particular case, I prefer to leave to my unconscious mind the task of creating a unique induction to fit this client's unique needs.

Trance is not synonym for being asleep; by the contrary, it is a state of high concentration in a reduced stimuli; it is a state of high responsiveness to suggestions.

Trance can be defined as a state in where intense communication is possible between a client and a practitioner. It happens all the time when two persons are discussing a very interesting subject, or a speaker deeply connects with an audience. Some church sermons are a pretty good example of this connection.

"Increased responsiveness occurs when attention is directed almost exclusively toward the patient, not when we are in a more self-centered state of mind"(Rosen, S. as mentioned in Zeig, J. 1994, p. 334).

The same author summarises the structure of trance and trance communication by adding that when a trance is attained, the barrier between the hypnotist and the subject is dissolved and the subject hears the hypnotist's voice as if it were coming from inside his or her own head.

"Any time a person focuses attention on one thing he will go into a trance" (Rosen S. Ibid). Erickson confirms this affirmation by adding, "Therapy consists of substituting a good idea for a bad idea." An example of a bad idea is the creation of self-fulfilling prophecies, i.e., "every time I am flying, I am getting a panic attack." It can be substituted by the affirmation . . . *It is very comfortable and it saves time to fly instead of driving.*

Notwithstanding this consideration, there are basic steps and principles that are at the base of the dynamic of trance. Some of them have been outlined in prior chapters:

Every client has contents, thoughts and experiences that can be identified by the therapist and included into the hypnotic message. Like most life events and experiences, they are not part of the client's awareness, but they can be elicited and utilized in the hypnotic trance to re-direct unconscious attention toward these events. We are to endeavour to teach the clients how to redirect their conscious and unconscious attention toward the events that are provoking ill health, via carefully crafted ambiguous statements.

We also have to keep in mind that the purpose of our intervention is to capture and direct the client's attention away from these events and re-direct and focus the attention toward the therapeutic message.

The Neo-Ericksonian School suggests these basic steps to be followed in the hypnotic sessions. (Walters, Havens 1993, p. 58-61).

1. Transition from an ordinary conversation into a hypnotic process

This is a procedure that has given me good results. I create the transition through depotentiating my client's conscious mind, and little by little inducing trance toward changework.

"Good morning John; It is nice meeting you (and) I will make sure that I am going to contact Dr. So-and-So to thank him for referring you to our office . . . (and) *I'm glad you decided to come to see me, because, when a person has a problem . . . and I assume you have a problem, it takes courage to come and see and talk with somebody they have never seen before . . . but seeing is believing . . . and you . . . truly believe that a problem can be solved . . . in any way, shape or form . . . and you can inform your unconscious mind . . . (Pacing their breathing) and your conscious mind . . . that there is a solution . . . and I don't know . . . and you don't know what that solution might be but your unconscious mind . . . which is the wisest part of you . . . already knows the solution . . . and you can access it . . . with your eyes open or closed . . . it is up to you . . . even though they are closing already . . . your eyelids down . . . going down . . . allowing every part of you . . . while breathing in and breathing out . . . to go into this dreamlike state . . . whenever you want to . . . taking your time . . . allowing your bodymind to relax . . . in a comfortable way.*

In here we intersperse a classical approach to create **fixation of attention** by focusing the client's attention on his inner reality, which will legitimize the trance. By responding to the client's emotional world, the induction's content becomes part of the client's inner self . . . *"John . . . I now know how difficult it is for you to accept the limitations, physical or otherwise that this pain of yours is creating . . . (and) I would like you to concentrate on this pain and . . . little-by-little . . . add a color and a shape to this pain . . . an inner feeling of discomfort (I again transform the pain into a "discomfort") that you can look at it . . . intensely . . . giving it a shape . . . a tri-dimensional shape that you can agree with . . . seeing it from the outside . . . looking at it . . . with ease . . . as if with a scientific curiosity . . . something that you can touch and shape as you see "fit" . . . while at the same time separating your individual self from the experience . . . giving it a purpose . . . while at the same time going deeper and deeper . . . into this new reality . . . a sudden comfort and calm . . . a deep feeling of relaxation . . . that explains and resolve any barriers that might interrupt the natural flow of things . . . feelings flowing like a river . . . cleansing everything . . . allowing you to just relax with the sound of water flowing down, down the slope . . . the gentle slope . . . as gentle as a dream that is produced when you close your eyes . . . and dream . . . That's right!*

2. Trance induction to capture and calm attention, and redirect it away from existing schemas or mental sets.

The statements of the trance induction are designed to capture the attention of clients and reassure and prepare them for their inner journey into the altered state of consciousness, also allowing them to detach from external stimulus . . . *and I don't know, and you don't know . . . the type of trance you want to achieve . . . perhaps a light trance . . . perhaps a deep trance . . . trance-forming thoughts . . . and intentions . . . and feelings and perceptions . . . into what you want to achieve today . . . and you can tell me . . . in your own time . . . in your own way . . . when your unconscious mind will*

*be ready for more learnings . . . allowing the rest of your body to rest
and relax . . . while your unconscious mind does the job . . . and when
your unconscious mind becomes ready . . . to let this comfortable trance
deepens . . . and I believe it wants to . . . it can bring the real issue . . .
which it will recognize . . . and let me know that it recognizes it . . . by
a slight motion of your right hand . . . at any time . . . your time . . .
That's right! . . . lifting your right hand . . . .*[21]

This redirection is also consonant with the classical
depotentiating of habitual frameworks and beliefs systems
suggested by Erickson, as a form of deepening the therapeutic
trance (Erickson and Rossi, 1996, p. 7). The use of surprise, shock,
distraction, or anything sudden or unexpected, interrupts the
client's habitual thought processes or habitual framework, thus
creating opportunities for reframing these processes or contents . . .
*Isn't amazing that an un-comfortable feeling is just a comfortable
feeling devoid of the "un" prefix? Something we construct in our mind
in the same way that we built or take away the addition of a house . . .
or a piece of furniture that we buy . . . and later on we give it away
to somebody . . . because we did not like it anymore? So many things
accumulated in the attic . . . waiting to be disposed of . . . to give
away . . . or take to the dump . . . a recycled gift given to somebody . . .
or donated . . . something that we have no use for . . . the flow of life
allowed to continue . . . every day . . . every month . . . every year.*

3. Metaphorical guidance and/or indirect suggestions that
stimulate unconscious search, understandings and responses.

Metaphors are used as a vehicle for teaching and exchanging
ideas. In my practice I noticed that it was easier to engage the
client's cooperation by immersing myself in his metaphorical world.
I realized that each client has amazing stories to tell and that these
stories can serve the purpose to re-create therapeutic tales that are
relevant to them.

Among northern First Nations people in Canada, as well as
among Ranqueles and Mapuche people in Argentina and Chile,

---

[21]   Ideomotor and Ideodynamic signals, created by Rossi and Cheek are methods
of accessing and resolving problems during therapeutic hypnosis.

storytelling is a gift that is truly respected. Dream tellers and Shaman use metaphors to convey Mores, Folkways and values to young people. Wisdom, in their cosmology, involves dreaming and storytelling.

A metaphor is a form of communication in which one event is conveyed in terms of an allegory to describe hidden or unnoticed aspect of what is being experienced. A problem situation can be expressed as if happening to a different person, creating the sensation that other person, not the client, might be going through similar experience. The intention is to depotentiate the client's fears about a personal experience or problem . . . a*nd I remember you telling me about your trip to the mountains . . . a beautiful mountain that you had to surmount . . . going down toward the river . . . and you cannot swim twice in the same river . . . which changes constantly . . . creating new life . . . cleansing others . . . keeping lives afloat . . . so many living things floating on water . . . their health afloat . . . your health afloat . . . floating away from mountains . . . creating new water ways; solving new and old problems . . . surmounting obstacles . . . cleansing the way down . . . feeling clean . . . comfortable . . . leaving behind . . . the load that cannot, should not . . . be carried . . .*

This step is also an opportunity for the client to peruse and thereafter utilize the content of his unconscious mind, which houses resources he normally does not know he possesses.

Metaphorical guidance and direct suggestions are the most organic forms of deepening a trance, by allowing the client to have control in exploring contents he already holds. Indirect suggestions are the most typical ways to allow this unconscious exploration, for they allow the client to have full responsibility of his processes . . . *wouldn't it be amazing to just allow something good to happen? Like walking in the park . . . one step after the other . . . allowing nature to fulfill its goals . . . allowing feeling to freely flow* (interspersal of an idea*) . . . allowing the unconscious transformation of thing . . . allowing the body to solve its own problems . . . in any way, shape or form . . . not even realizing that cells are created . . . tissue is replace . . . muscles are flexed . . .*

4. An opportunity for the participant to rehearse or practice new skills and attitudes.

The client assumes responsibility for the success of the therapeutic process. He feels empowered to rehearse new learnings obtained in the therapeutic meeting . . . *and I remember this story . . . of an elder camping with his grandchildren . . . at the end of a day talking around the fire . . . telling stories. In my head and my heart, he said . . . there are at any time two wolves fighting . . . . one representing everything that is good, . . . love . . . respect . . . loyalty . . . health . . . happiness . . . and the other representing everything that is bad . . . alcohol . . . laziness . . . envy . . . hate . . . fighting all the time . . . One of the grandchildren said to him . . . grandfather . . . whose wolf win? The grandfather answers . . . "**The one you feed**".*

5. Ending a Trance Session.

Since hypnosis is self-hypnosis and it is an interactive process, I let my clients know that it is up to them to choose the way and fashion in which they want to participate. When it is time to terminate the trance, and this has to be carefully calibrated, we close the final idea completely, leaving some posthypnotic commands for them to remember to . . . *go into a trance again . . . whenever you need to go into a trance . . .* I start bringing my client, little by little, back to the waking state, making sure that the transition is smooth and comfortable. They have to finish the session believing that it was a very, very positive experience they choose willingly to undertake. At this time, their unconscious mind will start rehearsing learnings obtained while in trance; . . . *and so . . . before you allow yourself to drift back to total awareness . . . you might give yourself the time to reflect . . . unconsciously . . . about the many learnings you may have obtained . . . The understandings . . . thoughts and images obtained . . . while your two minds interact; . . . unconscious learnings . . . that you can share with your conscious mind . . . reviewing those things that may need change or be replaced later on . . .*

6. Ratifying Trance

Trance ratification is incorporated into the process to make sure that the client is convinced that he underwent a state in which his unconscious world was accessed, providing him with an opportunity to be in contact with abilities he did not know he possessed . . . *and while you are preparing yourself to come out of this dreamlike state . . . you can use this time . . . to remember . . . the many learnings . . . that might have gone unnoticed by your conscious mind . . . but have been taken into consideration by your unconscious mind . . . while drifting up to the surface of consciousness . . . awakening . . . into a state of full awareness . . .*

Writing Hypnotic Scripts

I learnt from Ericksonian hypnotherapists that intuition is nothing more than the unconscious mind in action. Although I am convinced of the capabilities of the unconscious mind to recall stored information, I am also convinced that some of the interventions require a more specialized type of hypnotic scripts. Hence the need to create and develop a library of scripts that could address some of the most common problems and situations that clients bring into the therapist's office.

Writing scripts has to be one of the most challenging exercises of our profession. Milton Erickson, himself, spent a fair amount of time developing scripts for every occasion. One concept that resonates with me and which I consistently apply is the following:

When a client comes to me, or to any therapist's office, this client is suffering *today*; is seeking help *today for today's suffering*. Their pain does not have past or future, only present. We have to seize the moment and start right from where the client is. There is a precise time in which I have to touch his soul, listening carefully and with deep respect to what he is saying, for every one of his utterances are true to him, even if these statements are only the initial façade. This precise moment is a universe in itself and we have to become part of it.

From here on, it is going to be a journey together. Client and therapist becomes a unit in which the actors have different roles, but the roles are highly complementary. One cannot exist without the other and the client, by being who he is, qualifies and gives existence to the therapist.

The script has to reflect this precise moment and the theme has to be the client's theme.

Writing scripts does not happen in a vacuum. All my scripts are based in real cases and real experiences, or metaphors for real occurrences.

When a client is presenting a problem that resembles a prior situation in which some of the same elements were present, I search in my mind for the script and adapt it the best way I can to the situation, always thinking that my client may benefit from this experience.

The first step in writing a script is to search for sentences that describe the very present moment in which the client is positioned; physical position, such as sitting or reclined in a chair, sofa, etc., followed by the action the client is experiencing. I follow with descriptive statements of the situation and the circumstances that surround the client, as a way to add credibility to the initial statements (truisms).

E.g., . . . *you are in this room, sitting comfortably and relaxed . . . with your eyes closed . . . while wondering about the many things you may discover in the next minute . . . while surrounded by the sound of life around you . . . (car noises in the street).*

The second step is to insert a sentence that will allow the person to slowly accept a trance state, such as . . . *and you may notice that your muscles feel more and more relaxed . . . while your conscious mind thinks and imagine many things . . . even things that are not connected with what we are achieving here and now . . .* (because the mind wanders while I am attempting the induction, I must accept this reality) . . . (and) . . . *as your unconscious mind takes notes of what is happening around you . . . as you are giving yourself permission to experience these feelings of comfort and calm that makes* *your body heavier and heavier, while you are drifting down deeper and deeper . . .*

The third step is to alternate descriptive and suggestive statements while leading the client toward trance, interspersing sentences to assure him that he is safe, at the same time suggesting to give himself permission to get into a trance, e.g., . . . *and I am wondering, while you are in this safe place, how you will allow your unconscious mind to lead you into trance . . . and I do not know, and you do not know when it will be the precise time to . . . go into a trance, Now!*

The fourth step is to introduce metaphors that are relevant to the situation at hand, while attempting to keep the client unconsciously focused in the trance state.

During the whole process, we have to keep in mind that the attention fluctuates and that we have to remind the client constantly . . . *to go into a trance . . . and stay there.*

Once trance has been achieved, we introduce changework by adding direct suggestions for change. The therapist has to make sure that the suggestions have to be graduated to meet the goals of the meeting. It is very important to keep in the client's mind the notion that he or she is allowing his/her unconscious mind to find the answers he/she is seeking . . . *at any time, while you are going deeper and deeper into a dreamlike state . . . whenever the unconscious mind determines that it is convenient . . . and safe . . . to provide information and to integrate this knowledge into the conscious mind . . . unconsciously . . .*

The last step of writing scripts has to do with giving the client the space in which he will be able to return back into conscious awareness . . . (and) . . . *whenever you allow your unconscious mind to work on your behalf and to produce the answers that you are seeking . . . (and) whenever these answers are coming up into your unconscious mind . . . you will allow your conscious mind . . . to take its time in coming up to the surface, to a state of full awareness . . . in your own time . . . on your own way . . . opening your eyes . . . whenever you feel that is safe and comfortable to do so.*

It is recommended that when planning several meetings with the client, our scripts have to repeat the same ending to the process. This will allow the client to make adjustments and safely come back to the waking state.

I feel fortunate by having the possibility to work in both languages, English and Spanish. During my initiation as a therapist, my bilingual practice became a challenge because I was working with two sociological and linguistic realities, different values, different feelings, customs and expectations that cannot be translated into either language. This situation pressured me to use all my flexibility, imagination and ethical formation. This experience allowed me to work in a multidimensional, multicultural reality in which both worlds sometimes collided. In more than one occasion I needed desperately a script that would allow me to do the same, in English and in Spanish.

Hypnosis and Pain Control

While working with victims of the Chilean and Argentinean Military Coup, as well as in Canada with soldiers coming back from areas of conflict, I realized that under duress, the expression of pain and perception of pain changes in the presence of emotions intense enough to override pain nociception (pain reception). After living in Canada, I researched the mechanisms of pain modulation with the purpose of replicating the experience of analgesia and anaesthesia that seem to happen to persons undergoing undue pressure. In conjunction with this elemental form of analgesia and anaesthesia, an amnesia-like state evolves as a form of self-protection, for none of the victims were able to remember all the details of what took place, or the length in hours of the procedures. In a way the bodymind went into trance from the time in where war prisoners were placed a fabric bag in their heads[22] until the time they were released from the experience.

---

[22]   Covering the victim's head with a bag made of heavy fabric, or blindfolding the person seems to be a standard procedure in interrogations of this nature.

Another remarkable element connected with these types of situations is that under duress, the immune systems seems to work overtime to compensate the physical mistreatment, for few of the victims were suffering opportunistic sicknesses such as cold or infections.

While working with clients undergoing chemotherapy and radiation I discovered a connection between the amnesia-like state experienced by individuals suffering traumatic situations, like the shell shock type of reaction experienced by soldiers or war victims, and a similar phenomenon experienced by some of my clients undergoing these highly intrusive procedures, lengthy treatments, or a series of treatments, of which they forgot most of the details.

It is important to remark that the details of such events are no forgotten, but kept in our state-dependent memory bank, out of which they might surface in any situation having similar characteristic to the catastrophic events.

Like many people coming from politically unstable zones, I was in the past privy to information about traumatic situations, either by personal involvement or through my client's experiences. Sometimes this information surfaced under the most unusual conditions.

I was fortunate to be a patient of Dr. Roderick Morgan, an eye surgeon from Edmonton who pioneered many of the new surgical procedures for eye ailments. While undergoing cataracts and glaucoma laser treatment at the Royal Alexandra hospital, one of the physicians placed something on my head leaving exposed the area in where they were going to work. As soon as the lights were dimmed, my body went into an uncontrollable trembling, which made Dr. Morgan furious. "You have to trust your surgeon!!" (He stated angrily) "I cannot operate if you move"!

I had to request from him a space of time to explain about blindfolding and the shouting.

There was silence as he stated that he had never been exposed to these particular sorts of events. He immediately instructed his team to talk with me and describe the procedures, at the same time that they were talking about light events or making jokes. In the procedures that followed the initial one, he was carefully describing the process step-by-step. There was no trembling this time.

Because of the potential of similar situations happening to any practitioner (Canada has being a preferred destination for refugees from many countries), it is important to mention that, in the initial meetings with a client, we must search for state-dependent information that might have a bearing on results. Sometimes, while working with pain, experiences buried in the client's unconscious mind might come to the surface (abreaction), forcing the therapist to rapidly adapt to this new information. There might be, within the state-dependent memory, unconscious pain expressions creating unknown and hard to explain discomfort. I am equating unconscious pain with emotional or nonphysical pain or emotional distress.

Turk and Melzack established a distinction between primary nociceptive pain (caused by stimulation of pain receptors) and neuropathic pain (caused by an injury or dysfunction of peripheral or central nervous systems structures). (Turk D. Melzack R. 2001 p. 581).

I would like to add a third distinction, which is the emotional, psychological pain that sometimes is classified as idiopathic pain or originating from an unknown source.

In my experience as a practitioner working with cancer clients, this source might be the normal fear connected with a cancer diagnostic or with state-bound experiences believed to have some connection with the physician's diagnostic of cancer.

I noticed that sometimes my wife's unconscious mind, while she is deeply asleep, seems to connect with past memories of distress. Sometimes, while sleeping, she vocalizes her anger against an unknown stimulus. Years ago her vocalizations were in Spanish. Today, the same anger is expressed in English, which may indicate that, even if the unconscious memories were attained in one language, the acquisition of a new language does not change the contents. It changes only the languages in were they are expressed.

Forty years after our forced departure from Chile, these contents seem to remain intact.

I am of the impression that, in the case of a cancer diagnostic, the unconscious pain starts at the precise moment in where the physician informs the patient that he/she has a cancer condition. The state generated by this disclosure is similar to a hypnotic state and the memory of the event is learned immediately. From then on, it generates behaviors that might evolve into physical pain or unexplained fears.

Authors of the like of Herbert Spiegel have been equating this learning to the imprinting experienced by some mammals and birds. (Spiegel 1960 as mentioned by Rossi and Cheek, 1988, p 239-240). This imprinting-like process generates amnesia for the activating stimulus, compulsion to reproduce the imprinted reaction, and rationalization of the evoked behavior as a way to adapt to the new reality.

In many ways the experience suffered by clients undergoing chemotherapy mimics the traumatic experiences suffered by war victims. Some of them equated the process of receiving their chemical cocktail with a torture session. Mentally I agreed with them and I proceeded to incorporate their suffering into the hypnotic script. I customarily approach the treatment from two angles: Firstly, I use my personal experience to understand their fear of something being beyond their control, therefore concentrating in the present and projecting this present into the future as a way to rid the client of fear networks creating instead, through the use of age progression, an hopeful future. On occasions, while practicing in Chile, I ran into difficulty with the local medical association because, in their opinion, I was providing "false hopes" to the clients.

My second angle is to work in the present with the specific expression of pain. I concentrate on the symptoms, using pain amelioration and analgesia as convincers of the abilities and capabilities of the bodymind to problem-solve. I use scripts similar to this one:

"*Martha: I know that in the present you are undergoing chemotherapy and you want this process to be brief and over. Isn't it right? And I know that in your mind you want this to be over, and in your heart and soul this is something you truly, truly want. I know, as you know, that your bodymind, and my bodymind (establishing commonality) have capabilities beyond our comprehension. Our bodies are growing in every second of our existence and in each hour, each day, we produce new cells, new tissue and new experiences that makes us feel that time goes by without us knowing . . . but we know that we cannot stop time, and ten years from now* (I am already assuming that she will live at least ten more years) *you might think that all of these were some of the many obstacles a person has to overcome while growing old.*

That's right . . . if ten years went by, your view of the past (I am already positioning her ten years in the future **as if** she is already there) *is teaching you about how resilient your bodymind is . . . You are sixty years old now* (I am placing her ten years in the future), *ten years after you received treatment and . . . when looking back . . . you are able to visualize yourself receiving this treatment . . . and as I see my past . . . I can remember, as you can remember, how much you wanted to live your life . . . fulfill your purpose*" (I am creating an hopeful scenario ten years in the future, implying that this client is successfully controlling and eliminating her cancer). "*I remember my father growing old . . . and telling me about feeling the change of seasons on his bones . . . from summer to fall to winter . . . and me assuring him . . . that uncomfortable feelings like these are as strong as he perceived them* (I am avoiding to use the word pain). *Probably . . . by reducing these feelings in 10 per cent . . . you could make them more bearable . . . 90 percent being more tolerable than 100 percent . . . and when you reduce them in another ten percent . . . and you can do it as well Martha, . . . if you want to reduce them by ten percent . . . or in twenty percent . . . you can realize that eighty percent is more bearable . . . and you can give yourself this eighty percent, for it is you the one that controls your bodymind . . . that's right . . . but thirty percent will reduce the pain to a mere 70 percent, which is more bearable . . . is it not? That's right! 70 percent . . . allowing your body* *to be more flexible . . . more comfortable . . . while you are breathing in and out . . . in . . . and out . . . remembering how more comfortable it will be experiencing only sixty percent of it* (the pain) . . . *or fifty five . . . or fifty percent . . . as your bodymind rests and relax enjoying this reduction (and) . . . knowing that your bodymind can do it, as it did it the past, when you were a toddler . . . falling down every time you lost your balance* (Projecting the client toward an healthy past, when pain did not exist, thus reducing the memories of pain).

A sobering Experience

The day Freesia came into my office (see Freesia's case), I was forced to adapt to a very challenging case, in which a person perceived me as her last hope.

In order to generate in her the confidence that I could deliver something different, I had to work with her pain symptoms, while at the same time educating her about the workings of her bodymind.

On that precise day, I became a bona fide bilingual therapist.

I was forced, for the first time, to translate an English script directly into Spanish.

It was my first foray into pain amelioration in Spanish.

The book that I used as a guide was *Hypnosis for Change: A Practical Manual of Proven Hypnotic Techniques,* by Jossie Hadley and Carol Staudacher.

The script proved to be the one that cemented my professional relationship with this client. While I was translating it, Freesia was sitting comfortably in a chair in which her body was evenly supported, and her arms were comfortably relaxing in a wide armrest. Firstly, I concentrated in the pain in general to bring Freesia to the here-and-now. Then, little by little, I introduced the general induction for relaxation, followed by the induction for chronic pain. Once Freesia attained a deep trance, I followed with an induction for surgery, which is in fact, an induction for glove anaesthesia.

This is my translation of the Spanish induction:

I am glad that I can be of help to you, and I am truly thankful of you coming to see me. I believe that, by working together, we can produce changes that will make you feel better . . . and . . . better and . . . while you are accommodating in this chair, I would like you to give yourself permission to feel comfortable . . . and . . . in order for you to be comfortable . . . you can adjust your body to this chair . . . any time you want . . . and I know . . . and you know . . . that we work with two minds . . . your unconscious mind . . . and your conscious mind . . . and one is more intelligent that the other . . . and you are . . . right now . . . allowing your unconscious mind . . . to guide you in this experience . . . and your conscious mind and your unconscious mind . . . both of them in one unit . . . know that you have an uncomfortable situation . . . an uncomfortable feeling . . . **but** *. . .* (I used here the word "but" to establish a need to change her feelings) *what a joy it is to know that uncomfortable feelings . . . can become comfortable feelings . . . by simply knowing that everything changes continuously . . . and you can feel comfortable . . . with your eyes closed or open . . . It is up to you to decide in which way . . . you will* **go into a trance** *. . . little . . . by . . . little . . . allowing your body to become heavier and heavier . . . and your arms to feel heavier and heavier, resting comfortably . . . on your chair . . . and you are deeper . . . and deeper feeling more and more relaxed . . .* **are you not?**

(Freesia assented with her head) *. . . and as you are feeling more and more relaxed and comfortable . . . your unconscious mind is telling you that you are in a safe place . . . safe to experience any change to these uncomfortable feelings you might desire.*

(I am avoiding using the word "pain") *. . . That's right . . . allowing your body . . . your right arm . . . your left arm . . . your right leg . . . and your left leg . . . to feel comfortable and relaxed . . . and I would like you to give yourself permission to focus your attention . . . consciously . . . and unconsciously . . . on your uncomfortable feelings (pain) . . . eliminating the dark cloud over your head . . . floating away, little by little first . . . and faster and faster as the wind pushes them away . . . away from over your head . . . away from this place . . . dissolving in the wind of the south . . . the gentle wind that brings to* *us the blue sky . . . and the light of the sun that makes everything so different . . . so soothing . . . caressing the plants and the trees and the people . . . touching us . . . making us alive and well to enjoy the gentle breeze of the south . . . making everything seem happier . . . and calmer . . . and healthier . . . a gentle breeze . . . a gentle feeling of comfort . . . **that's right!** . . . ready to do what it takes . . . to feel well . . . to feel good . . . to feel free.*

(I went right away into an induction for pain amelioration and control, to reinforce the notion that she had the tools to control pain).

Now I want you to focus your attention on one of your hands . . . and begin to imagine that hand becoming numb . . . recalling a time when your hand fell asleep . . . and how wooden your hand felt . . . and as you purposefully numb your hand . . . imagine a tingling beginning in your fingertip . . . and a warm feeling flowing through your hand . . . and soon all feelings will drain out of your hand; . . . all feelings draining away . . . while you are allowing these wooden, leathery feelings to irradiate all over that hand. Now let that hand to be numb . . . to stay numb . . . completely numb. Let all these feelings on your fingertips go to your wrist . . . and drain out of your hand . . . let everything drain out of your hand . . . this numbness spreading out . . . draining out of your hand . . . those feelings of numbness increasing and spreading out . . . and while your mind concentrates on that numb hand . . . you can feel yourself sleeping safely, gently . . . deeply . . . into a level of total relaxation . . . Just letting these feelings of relaxation and numbness to increase . . . feeling so numb . . . soooo relaxed!

Your hand is now totally numb . . . completely numb . . . and you can feel this numbness in your hand . . . which now travels towards the part of your body that feels the discomfort . . . gently touching it . . . and making it numb . . . allowing the numbness of your hand to spread (the numbness) *all over your lower abdomen . . .* (I inserted the part of Freesia's body that was in pain. Freesia moved her hand in circular, slow motion covering the zone) *. . . over that part that you want to be numb . . . and let the numbness drain out of your hand and into your lower abdomen . . . NOOOW! Feel your abdomen* *becoming numb . . . wooden . . . heavy . . . numb . . . numb and thick as if it were made of wood . . . and when all the numbness has left your hand . . . place your hand back down into a comfortable position . . . keeping your abdomen numbed for as long as you need to . . . as long as you want to . . . (and) when you have completed a total numbness . . . just let it go and feel the numbness drain away . . . draining taking away the uncomfortable feelings . . . your abdomen returning to normal . . . and you can use your time now . . . while you are still allowing your unconscious mind to keep you in a trance . . . to reflect . . . unconsciously on the very moment in which your unconscious mind allowed you to feel better and better, and in how this feeling of comfort extends . . . beyond your unconscious mind . . . and into your conscious mind . . . providing relief . . . for as long as you want to . . . **That's right!** . . . take some time now . . . to review the experience . . . and extend it into the level of awareness . . . and whenever you feel that you want to open your eyes . . . whenever you want to drift back to total awareness . . . you can keep this feeling of numbness . . . for as long as you want . . . feeling awake . . . feeling well . . . feeling good . . . That's right! Opening your eyes any time . . . now. (Adapted from Hadley and Staudacher, pgs.190-191).*

This Spanish translated induction was very effective, allowing Freesia to learn how to control her pain. Her most important learning was that she had a conscious mind, and an unconscious mind, and that both minds were working on her behalf. Her second learning was that she had control over her body and that this control was available to her at any time.

The Hadley and Staudacher induction allowed me to use it as a prompting, a base to create a proximal Spanish version to create the desired numbness. Later on, it became easier for me to provide glove anaesthesia without a script, by utilizing information produced by the client. To be proficient in the use of the technique, I memorized it and extended it by adding some elements coming from the client's experience, while keeping its integrity. This particular induction proved to be very effective any time I used it with people suffering pain. As for Freesia, she learned to use it beyond the confines of the office. Many times she asked me over the telephone to provide the induction, especially when she felt unable to reproduce the desired results.

Working with Pain: Specific Considerations; The Use of Switches in Pain Amelioration

Pain is not always a simple, disagreeable, nasty stimulus. It is a complex construct with temporal, emotional, psychological and somatic expressions, many of them not amenable to chemical treatment. In Dr. Milton Erickson's words, the pain experience is composed of past-remembered pain, of present pain experience, and of anticipated pain of the future. Immediate pain is augmented by past pain and is enhanced by the future possibility of pain (Rossi 1980, p. 238–244); therefore, fear is connected with the possible pain of the future.

I am of the opinion that pain is what brings a client to the practitioner. Pain is evident in every consultation and it represents not only the physical expression, but also the more encompassing emotional suffering manifested as depression, anxiety, phobias, etc.

A form of pain is therefore contained in any problem expressed by a suffering client. It requires, above all, comfort and understanding, and the role of the practitioner is to identify, together with the suffering client, the way in which it is manifested. Alleviation or amelioration of pain is what is at the center of therapy.

Following this all-encompassing philosophy, I tend to concentrate mostly in pain amelioration. I customarily stay away from its total abolition, for it is difficult to achieve and, if failing, it might destroy the trust deposited on the capabilities of the professional. I rather utilize an indirect, permissive approach to pain abolition that leaves the control of outcome to the client. I tend to favour the use of switches to redirect and alter pain perception. Images, past positive experiences, voice inflexion, therapeutic tales, metaphors and colors, can be utilized as switches.

If we accept that reality is not what it is but what is perceived, we can also accept that, because perceptions can be changed, reality as a perceived by the client can be altered, can be switched into something else.

By creating a positive state of mind, we can "switch" or substitute the negative pain experience for a positive state. This is called, of course, a positive switch, i.e. the expression . . . *"Every time fall approaches, I feel a sense of doom and my entire body starts aching and my joints swelling because of humidity"* . . . can be switched by commenting about "the amazing capability of nature to decorate every tree with leaves of every color".

Identifying negative switches will give us the opportunity to intervene, to block negative thoughts by offering alternative images or thoughts. Sometimes changing or eliminating words would ameliorate the perception of pain. I.e. substituting the word pain for the expression "bothersome feeling" or "uncomfortable feeling" takes the edge of pain. As the reader already know, every time we mention the word "pain", we remind the client of his suffering, bringing to the fore all its attributes, therefore the word "pain" must not be mentioned.

John . . . I remembered you phoning me and explaining me the nature of your problems, (and) I must tell you that what you are bringing to the office is quite a burden, but burden is a weight that can be lifted, and I am aware that in your job in the oil patch you have lifted all sorts of weights . . . (I am switching and diluting the pain into a burden and further transforming it into a weight, which can be interpreted in many forms, not strictly connected with "pain"). *As you already know, in this office we transform (trance-form) all sorts of experiences and I would like you to give yourself the opportunity to research all the areas that in your opinion we should explore . . . with the purpose of changing them . . . (and) as you already know, WCB (Workers compensation Board) sent us a list of your physical problems as well as a listing of the feelings that in their opinion you have attached to the problem* (the word "feeling" is encompassing of all expressions of pain, but it has a lesser emotional connotation.

Since pain is a construct composed of past, present and future pain, I am attempting to divide the experience of pain in three sections therefore reducing the pain in thirds.) . . . (and) as *mentioned in your file, you fell from a ladder about two years ago . . . .would you please tell me where were you two years ago . . . ?*
By the way . . . where were you and your family two years ago? (I am attempting to take him to the past to search for pleasant memories to switch the past experience of pain. I also pause to give him the opportunity to tell me about his family) . . . *I was also informed that you were a very good hockey player . . . and hockey is a rough sport with lots of opportunities to injure yourself or injuring the opposite player . . .* (hockey is the national sport in Canada. It requires speed and physical strength, with ample opportunities for the players to receive injuries, but it is what some players call a good and satisfying pain) . . . *are there any one of your children interested in the sport?* (I am attempting to introduce another procedure for hypnotic control of pain, which is the creation of amnesia. By concentrating on a subject totally disconnected from the experience of pain, a person tends to forget his/her pain).

(John started recalling the times in where he played hockey and that his children were avid hockey players dreaming of a future in the NHL) . . . .

(When dealing with pain, and when the need to use multiple approaches to pain management becomes apparent, I carefully connect the previous procedure with the new one, thus eliminating the possibility for the client to go back into the experience of pain. In order to connect procedures, I attempt to empower the client with control over the flow, allowing him to own the whole process) . . . *"And as you go back and forth, remembering those pleasant memories . . . allowing your bodymind to remember how well you dealt with unpleasant experiences . . . transforming the day . . . the night . . . the next day . . . in just a part and parcel of what you are* (I am switching to a present time) . . . *what you want to be . . . what you want to feel . . . feeling this tingling sensation on the tip of your fingers . . . moving upward toward the elbow . . . doing it your way . . . taking your time . . . allowing the feeling to spread all over your arm . . . a pleasant feeling of numbness . . . decreasing the feeling . . . a little bit at a time . . . the sensation flowing out of your arm . . . a lesser feeling when touched . . . reducing it in a percentage..90 percent down . . . or perhaps 80 percent . . . feeling the numbness to spread . . . in a 70 or perhaps 60 percent . . . counting down . . . allowing your unconscious mind to take over . . . a 50 percent of reduction to the touch . . . a soft and decreasing feeling . . . a wooden feeling to the touch . . . a comfortable feeling flowing away from your arm . . . that's right . . . allowing your arm to become numb to the touch . . . feeling nothing.* (Here I touch the arm toward the hand, to check the progressive numbness, assuming and allowing the client to assume that it is in fact numb to the touch).

Throughout the procedure, the practitioner's body language must communicate to the client that the numbness and analgesia is happening, is taking place and success is assured. Sometimes a procedure called fractionation or fractional approach can be used to train the client to achieve analgesia, by bringing the client in and out of the procedure, each time going deeper into the experience, until he becomes accustomed to the trance state.

It is essential to understand that the different interpretations of the pain experience will determine the hypnotic approach to be used. Erickson states that *"each interpretation leads to differing psychological frameworks- to varying ideas and associations"* . . . which will determine the most effective hypnotic procedure to be utilized to ameliorate pain. (Erickson, M. MD, 1992, p. 222)

In concluding, it is important to remember that the antidote to pain is to unblock pain paralysis by empowering the client with the notion that he possesses, within his bodymind, options beyond the chemical ones. Bandler and Grinder remind us that every human being in his life cycle has transition-crisis points; some individuals are able to negotiate these periods of change with little difficulty, whereas some others, in front of similar crisis, see these points as periods of dread and pain. The difference between the two groups is that the people responding creatively and exhibiting more stress-solving skills are the ones capable of perceiving a wider range of options to choose from.

"The most pervasive paradox of the human condition . . . is that the processes which allow us to survive, grow, change, and experience joy, are the same processes which allow us to maintain an impoverished model of the world" (Bandler, Grinder, J. 1975, p. 13-14).

Additional techniques for pain control will be discussed in a different volume totally dedicated to this phenomenon. Pain, perception of pain and techniques for its treatment requires a volume of its own.

EPILOGUE

As of today, November 05, 2014, my wife and I we have lived with Cancer for almost thirty years. In an interesting conversation, our oncologist commented on the fact that humankind have tried unsuccessfully to eliminate cockroaches and ants for centuries, until they resolved to "live with", not to "fight" these insects considered nuisances. As a strange parallel, we have lived with cancer for all these years, switching from concentrating our lives on fighting cancer, to dedicating our time to personal and professional growth. When cancer comes, and it has come three times, we concentrate on the present using all the tools we possess to resolve it. Sometimes, the idea that she is on stage four (a thirty-year-old cancer is a stage four cancer) cross our mind. We have learned that actually these stages are statistics that in no way encroaches on our life meaning and purposes.

Since Matty's immune system is working well, we trust that the next examination will produce the same unremarkable results she has produced for the last 29 years.

Many years ago Matilde learned about using imagery and self-hypnosis to improve the functioning of her immune system. For almost three decades she has been using her training to consciously program her unconscious mind for success. Even though the old fears manage to partially come back on the days prior to her routine examinations, she is a "living" proof that her system works.

As for my experience as a Psycho-Oncologist and hypnotherapist I am of the opinion that working the maps of the mind, and placing the client, not the sickness at the center of therapy, is the most suitable way to incorporate this client into the healing process. I learned vicariously that healing is self-healing.

In spite of the works of a myriad of practitioners, the medical establishment is still timid in assigning hypnosis its rightful place.

While perusing all the books on pain control at the library of the University of Alberta in Edmonton, I found a book titled *Psychology, Pain, and Anaesthesia* edited by H. B. Gibson. It was apparently the only book available to medical school students, which had a chapter dedicated to hypnotic techniques in pain control. The chapter was brief and light in content, describing in few details the work of Spiegel and Spiegel and Hilgard and Hilgard. It briefly described some techniques for pain amelioration by Barber and Erickson, finally giving hypnosis a passing grade as a technique for symptomatic relief of pain, while carefully qualifying its effectiveness in the absence of exploratory methods and assessments, such as the Beck Anxiety Inventory, and the Beck Depression Inventory, which in my opinion have no psychometric connections with the trance state.

I am of the impression that we are still a long ways away from full acceptance of hypnosis and trance states as a legitimate tool for emotional and physical healing. I hope my effort will create some interest in perusing these healing tools even further.

I was surprised by the emphasis that a school of the calibre of the Harvard School of Medicine placed on Meditation. It allowed me to understand why the Inspire Health Clinic in Vancouver initiates the day guiding patients and staff in a morning meditation exercise.

Ajahn Amaro, a Buddhist monk, while defining Dukkha (suffering–dissatisfaction), equated this state with dissatisfaction, with the capacity of the mind to lose its balance, thus becoming emotionally stressed. In solving Dukkha, he mentions the Four Noble Truth. He equated these noble Truths to a medical diagnosis.

Dukkha, or dissatisfaction is the symptom.

The Second Element describes what is causing Dukkha; self-centered craving, greed, hatred, and delusion, negative afflicting emotions, habits and qualities contained in the mind poisoning the heart.

The Third Element is the prognosis, which in Ajahn Amaro's teachings is always curable. The experience of dissatisfaction can end because we have the capacity to free ourselves from it.

The Fourth Element is the methodology of treatment, the way in which we heal the wound: responsible behavior, living an ethical and moral life, mental collectedness, meditation and mind training, and lastly, development of insightful understanding in accordance with reality, or wisdom.

The comment that affected me the most was that there are two levels of Dukkha, two dimensions of the experience of dissatisfaction: The first one is the experience of physical and emotional pain. The second element is what Ajahn Amaro calls Adventitious suffering, or what the mind adds to a negative experience, represented by the fretfulness, resistance, resentment, and anxiety we create around the experience.

It is clear to me now that our role as therapists is to find meaning in pain, to explain what lies behind this experience, and then meditate on the nature of the experience, dissociating ourselves from it and looking at it with an inquisitive mind devoid of judgment. Meditation is the innate capacity of the mind to investigate, explore and contemplate the nature of the experience, materialized in the act of focusing our attention in a meditation object, like our breathing, with the intention of training our mind to focus in the present, and . . . "Learning how to think when we choose to think, and learning how not to think when we choose not to . . ." (Kabat-Zinn 2011, pp.31–33)

This opens the door to the use of the ultimate capacity of the mind, to investigate and to understand life experiences, to learn how to separate from Dukkha, and to focus on what is truly, truly important.

REFERENCES

1. Ader, Robert, et al. (1990). *Psychoneuroimmunology*. San Diego, Academic Press.
2. *BBC1 Health Magazine*. September 30, 2002.
3. Bandler, Richard (2008). *Richard Bandler's Guide to Trance-formation*. HCI, Florida.
4. Bandler, Richard and Grinder, John. (1975) "The Structure of Magic" SBB, Inc. Palo Alto, California.
5. Blass, Thomas., PhD. (1968). *The Man Who Shocked the World*. Basic Books.
6. Black, Max. (1968) *The Labyrinth of Language*. Mentor Books.
7. CONILE (2003) Comisión Nacional de Ayuda al Niño Leucémico. Santiago, Chile.
8. Chopra, Deepak (2002). *The Deeper Wound*. Harmony Book.
9. Chomsky, Noam (1968) *Language and Mind*. Harcourt Brace.
10. Dacher, Elliott, MD (1991) *PNI. The New Mind/Body Healing Program*. Paragon House.
11. Dienstfrey, Harris. (1991) *Where the Mind Meets the Body*. Harper Collins Publishers.
12. Divine, Laura (2009) *Journal of Integral Theory and Practice*. A Post disciplinary Discourse for Global Action. Spring 2009. Integral Institute. Boulder. CO.
13. Erickson, Milton (1965) "An introduction to the study and application of hypnosis in pain control," Seminar given in Seattle, Washington, May 21-23.
14. Erickson, Milton. and Rossi, Ernest. (1996) "Experiencing Hypnosis" *Therapeutic Approaches to Altered States*. Irvington Publishers.

15. Erickson, Milton and Rossi, Ernest. (1996) *"Hypnotherapy: An Exploratory Casebook."* Irvington Publishers.
16. Erickson, Milton. (1992) *Healing in Hypnosis.* Irvington Publishers.
17. Fisher, Erik. (1997) Private correspondence. Email letter to EricksonList@topica.com
18. Fordyce, Fowler, et al. (1973) *"Operant Conditioning in the treatment of chronic Pain."* Arch. Phys.Med. 1. The Lancet.
19. Frankl, Viktor (1984) *"The Unheard Cry for Meaning,"* Washington Square Press.
20. Fricchione, Gregory. (2011). Notes from the *"Revolutionary Mind/Body Medicine"* seminars. Harvard Medical School. October 2011.
21. Gilligan, Stephen. (1987) *"Therapeutic Trances."* The Cooperation Principle in Ericksonian Hypnotherapy." Brunner Rutledge.
22. Glaser, William, MD (1984) *"Control Theory"*. Harper & Row.
23. Gordon, James., MD (1996) *"Manifesto for a New Medicine."* Your Guide for Healing Partnership and the Wise Use of Alternative Therapies. Perseus Books.
24. Gordon, David. (1978) *"Therapeutic Metaph*ors." Meta Publications.
25. Greene, Judith. (1973) *"Psycholinguistics."* Chomsky and Psychology. Penguin Books.
26. Grof, Stanislav (2000) *"Psychology of the Future"* . . . SUNY Series.
27. Hersen, Michael., Biaggio, Maryka. (2000) *"Effective Brief Therapy"* A Clinician's Guide. Academic Press. N.Y.
28. Havens, Ronald (1985). *The Wisdom of Milton H. Erickson.* Irvington Publishers.
29. Hendley, Steven (1956). *"From Communicative Action to the Face of the Other."* Levinas and Habermas on Language Obligation and Community. Lexington Books.
30. Hadley Josie. Staudacher, Carol. (1985) *"Hypnosis for Change."* A Practical Manual of Proven Hypnotic Techniques. Ballantine Books.

31. Havens, Ronald. Walters, Catherine. (1989) *"Hypnotherapy Scripts"*. *A Neo-Ericksonian Approach to Persuasive Healing*. Brunner Mazel.

32. Holland. Jimmie, Rowland Julia Howe, Eds. (1989) *"Handbook of Psycho-Oncology"* New York Oxford University Press.

33. Holland, Jimmie.C. et al. *Psycho-Oncology,* 2nd.Ed. Oxford University Press 2010.

34. *Journal of the American Medical Association*.1992.

35. Jackendoff, Ray (1999) *"Languages of the Mind."* Essays on *Mental Representations*. MIT Press. 1999.

36. James, Tad. Flores, Lori and Schober, Jack. (2000) *"Hypnosis. A comprehensive Guide"*. *Producing Deep Trance Phenomena*. Crown House Publishing.

37. Kabat-Zinn Jon (1990) *"Full Catastrophe Living"* Delta Books.

38. Kabat-Zinn Jon, Davidson, Richard (2011) *"The Mind's Own Physician"*. *A Scientific Dialogue with the Dalai Lama on the Healing Power of Meditation*. Mind and Life Institute. New Harbinger Publications Inc. CA.

39. Lankton, Stephen. and Lankton, Carol. (1983) *"The Answer Within: A Clinical Framework of Ericksonian Hypnotherapy"* Brunner Mazel, N.Y.

40. *Mindbody Medical Institute Journal*. September 18.2002.

41. Moyers, Bill. (1993) *"Healing and the Mind"*. Doubleday.

42. Melzack, Ronald. (1998) *"Pain and stress: A new perspective*. New York Gilford Press.

43. Turk Dennis. and Melzack Ronald. (2001) *"Handbook of Pain Assessment, Second Edition."* The Gilford Press, N.Y.

44. Milgram, Stanley. (1969) *"Obedience to Authority"*. *An Experimental View*. Perennial Classics.

45. Mindell. Arnold PhD. (2004). *"The Quantum Mind and Healing"* Hampton Roads Publishing Co. Inc. Charlottesville. VA.

46. Pecarve, Reuben. (2002) *"The Hypnosis Book."* How to use *Hypnotic Techniques to Improve Physical and Mental Health*. Optimum Publishing International. Montreal

47. Parham, Peter. (2000) *"The Immune System."* Garland Publishing.

48. Rabow, M. and McPhee, S. Edmonton Journal, November 25, 2002.

49. Rossi, Ernest L. (1986). *"The psychobiology of Mindbody Healing"* W.W. Norton & Co.

50. Rossi, Ernest, Cheek, David B. (1988) *"Mindbody Therapy."* Methods of Ideodynamic Healing in Hypnosis. W.W. Norton &Co.

51. Rossi Ernest (1980) *"The Collected Papers of Milton Erickson MD. Vol. IV"* Irvington Publishers N.Y.

52. Rossi, Ernest (1991) *"The 20 Minute Break."* Tarcher. Los Angeles.CA.

53. Simonton, Carl MD, et al. (1992) *"Getting Well Again."* Bantam Books.

54. Selye, Hans (1956) *"The Stress of Life."* McGraw-Hill Book Company Inc.

55. Siegel, Bernie (1998) *"Love, Medicine, and Miracles."* Harper Perennial.

56. Spiegel, Herbert and Spiegel, David (1978) *"Trance and Treatment."* Basic Books, N.Y.

57. Sternberg, Esther, MD. (2000) *"The Balance Within."* The Science Connecting Health and Emotions. W.H. Freeman and Co.

58. Selby, John and Von Luhmann, Manfred, MD. (1989) *"Conscious Healing".* Visualizations to boost your Immune System. Bantam New Age Books.1989.

59. Singh-Khalsa, Dharma MD and Stauth, Cameron. (1999) *"The Pain Cure"* The Proven Medical Program that Helps End Chronic Pain. Warner Books.

60. Stiefel, Friedrich. (2006) *"Communication in Cancer Care."* 2006. Springer-Verlag Heidelberg.

61. Weinstein, Eugenia, et al. (1987). *"Trauma, Duelo y Reparación. Una experiencia de trabajo psicosocial en Chile."* Fasic-Editorial Interamericana.

62. Tart, Charles. (1969) *"Altered States of Consciousness".* A Doubleday Anchor Book.

63. Themes, Roberta (1999) *"Medical Hypnosis" An introduction and Clinical Guide.* Harcourt Brasse.

64. Turk, Dennis and Melzack, Ronald. (2001) *Handbook of Pain Assessment.* Second Edition. Guilford Press.

65. Vanderhaegue, Lorna and Bouic, Patrick (2002) *"The Immune System Cure".* Prentice Hall Canada.

66. World Health Organization. *Technical Report Series 804, Cancer Pain, and Palliative Care.* Geneva: World Health Organization 1990:11.

67. Walters, Catherine. and Havens, Ronald. (1993) *"Hypnotherapy for Health, Harmony and Peak Performance."* Expanding the Goals of Psychotherapy. Brunner Mazel.

68. Wilber, Ken (2000) *"Grace and Grit" Spirituality and Healing in the Life and Death of Treya Killam Wilber.* Shambhala Boston.

69. Wilber, Ken (1998) *"The Marriage of Sense and Soul."* Integrating Science and Religion. Random House Inc. N.Y.

70. Wilber, Ken. (2000) *"Integral Psychology." Consciousness, Spirit, Psychology, Therapy.* Shambhala, Boston.

71. Wilson, Timothy. (2002) *"Strangers to Ourselves."* Belknap Harvard Cambridge.

72. Yapko, Michael (1997) *"Breaking the Patterns of Depression."* Doubleday N.Y.

73. Zeig, Jeffrey. (1994) *"Ericksonian Methods"" The Essence of the Story.* Brunner-Mazel. N.Y.